A few words about the
columnist who's been called...

> —a sexy Dear Abby,
> —a bawdy Miss Manners,
> —a hipper Dr. Ruth,
>   *and*
> —The Ann Landers of Lust:

"Isadora Alman is chicken soup for the sexually bewildered, an erotic cornucopia for inquiring minds who need to know, and a true queen among queens. Isadora's is the first page San Francisco turns to; thousands of San Franciscans owe a debt to Ms. Alman's warm and understanding heart."
—Elgy Gillespie,
Editor, *San Francisco Review of Books*

"Funny, dirty and true."
—Alice Kahn, *San Francisco Chronicle*

"Unlike those twin relics of the repressive forties and fifties, Abigail Van Buren and Ann Landers, Isadora Alman is always entertaining, hilarious, and she doesn't kvetch."
—Maitland Zane, *San Francisco Chronicle*

"Isadora is sharp, witty, fresh and authentic when it comes to love and sex. We sexologists rate Alman as one of our best."
—Dr. Sol Gordon, former director, Institute for Family Research and Education

"Reading Isadora Alman's book, like making love, will teach you many strange and wonderful things about yourself and other people. And like good sex, reading Isadora is an experience that could become habit-forming."
—Jeremy Klein, Editor, *Et cetera* (the journal of the International Society for General Semantics)

"Isadora is a first-rate sex communicator. Her intelligence, humor, and generosity nurture the erotic potential in all of us."
—Betty Dodson, author of *Sex for One*

"'Did you read what Isadora said today?' is heard often in San Francisco and New York—and for good reason. She is witty, outrageous, and courageous. The big bonus is, Isadora gives great (and important) facts, sorely needed in this sexually suspicious and reactionary time. For a good time, and a thorough education, you've got to read this book."
—Dr. Tina Tessina, therapist; author of *How to Be a Couple and Still Be Free*

"Isadora Alman's writing is terrific—witty yet empathetic, informative, entertaining."
—Marc and Judith Meshorer, co-authors of *Ultimate Pleasure: The Secrets of Easily Orgasmic Women*

"I would rather people said Dr. Ruth is a Germanic Isadora Alman."
—Isadora Alman

ask isadora

**Collected Columns
on Sex and
Relationships
from
*The San Francisco
Bay Guardian***

by
isadora alman

ASK ISADORA

Copyright © 1991 by Masquerade Books, Inc.
All Rights Reserved

No part of this book may be reproduced, stored in a retrieval system, or transmitted in any form, by any means, including mechanical, electronic, photocopying, recording, or otherwise, without prior written permission from the publisher.

First Masquerade Books Edition 1991

First Printing September 1991

ISBN 1-878320-61-0

Cover design by Steve Powell

Printed in the United States of America
Published by Masquerade Books, Inc.
801 Second Avenue
New York, N.Y. 10017

*To those I love
and those who love me:*

*Satisfying communication
is much of the reason why.*

Contents

Foreword by Maitland Zane		9
Introduction		*11*
1	A Rose by Any Other Name: Terminology	15
2	The Way It's Supposed to Be: Myths, Beliefs, and Expectations	33
3	Conversations with Oneself: Clarifying Issues	53
4	And All the Flesh Is Heir To: Bodies	67
5	Fantasy and Friction: Solo Sex	101
6	The Opposite Sex: Men/Women	111
7	Without Unwanted Consequences: Sexually Transmitted Conditions	125
8	The Social Squaredance: Meeting, Mingling, and Finding Partners	143
9	Communication Is the Best Lubrication: Communication Techniques	167
10	Negotiating a Relationship	191
11	Exotica	215
12	Resources and Research	231
About the Author		*255*

Foreword
by Maitland Zane

The posture is preposterous, the pleasure transitory...and yet, is there anything more important in life than making the beast with two backs? In Isadora Alman's case, perhaps three or four, and that's what makes her the only sex-advice columnist I know who can explore the frontiers of sex without sounding like a sniggering voyeur, or worse yet a pontificating shrink.

Those of us who dwell on the lunatic fringe of the continent have been reading her columns for the past several years in the *San Francisco Bay Guardian*, sometimes if we're lucky catching her warm radio voice. Isadora is always entertaining and often hilarious. What is her secret? For me, at least, an acceptance of the myriad complexities of human sexuality. Unlike Abigail Van Buren and Ann Landers, those twin relics of the repressive Forties and Fifties, she doesn't kvetch, she doesn't wag her finger, and she doesn't fall back on the tired formula, "seek professional help."

Unlike the superannuated nymphomaniacs of the stroke magazines, Ms. Alman's intent is not prurient. She's heard it all, the reader feels. She's been around the track of love and lust, there's nothing one could say (or write) that would shock her; she even has a kind word for bondage freaks and enema addicts.

In literary terms, one can look back to Nathanael West's troubling novel *Miss Lonelyhearts*, but many will also see her as a worthy successor to Eugene ("Dr. Hip") Schoenfeld,

M.D., who had a sex-and-drugs column in the *Berkeley Barb* more than twenty years ago.

What makes Ms. Alman so readable is her mix of the serious and the frivolous. I'm thinking of her recent tongue-in-cheek report on that movie star who, the gossip went, allegedly lets declawed gerbils crawl up his backside. Isadora might even teach you a new word or two...*vart,* for instance: a vaginal fart. The word was coined by one of her many fans, a beautiful Brit we'll call Susan Priest.

But who is Isadora in real life? A straight lady who lives in a cosy house in San Francisco's Richmond district, a woman who has an open relationship with her mate but has chosen monogamy. Isadora Alman would make a great ringmistress at a wild party. I can see her now, serving goodies and drinks, stepping lightly over cavorting couples with the line, "That's right, kids, don't fight."

Introduction

Recently I was sitting in the waiting room of a physician who runs a family practice. Near me was a young mother trying to amuse the squirming toddler on her lap. "What's this?" she pointed. "Nose! That's right. Good for you. And what's this?" Prolonging the inventory as far as she could, she tenderly poked and queried her way down the baby's body, to their mutual delight. "This?" asked the baby, taken over his mother's role. "That's your belly button." "This?" the little one said, reaching the inevitable.

There is an expression from the Deep South about genteel folk who "wouldn't say 'shit' if they had a mouthful." My father used to joke about giving baby Isadora a bath, during which he would wash as low as possible and as high as possible, but I would have to wash Possible myself. Now, fortymumble years later, in my professional capacity I can, with nary a blush, give you many names, from street slang to clinical Latin, for every aspect of genital minutiae. On my own body in off-duty hours, however, I possess a "down there."

"This? This?" the toddler was demanding and pointing into his lap. The rhythm of the game was interrupted by Mother's growing pause. I awaited the young woman's response as eagerly as the squirming baby.

"Why don't we read about Babar now?" she suggested. Grabbing the topmost book off the play table by her side. "Do you want to hear about the elephant?"

And here we have it—another therapy client

in the making who, in adulthood, is going to wonder why she or he finds sex so problematic when "it ought to be a perfectly natural method of self expression" ...*And* each of us should be able to find a complimentary Other, love should transform us all, and living happily ever after be the order of the day, right?

We are all shaped by our upbringing, our times, and the prevailing myths of the advertising industry. The indoctrination of cultural beliefs is all-pervasive, from childhood fairy tales to today's musical Top Forty. It requires careful vigilance not to swallow it whole, painstaking sorting-through and spitting-out to avoid being sickened by it.

Even though this collection of columns has been edited to reduce repetition—(I receive at the very least one question about penis size, and two or three about finding partners, in every week's mail)—you will notice that certain soon-recognizable erroneous beliefs underlie many of the questions represented here. These are:

1.) There is one right way for a relationship to be, and somehow you were absent from school the day they handed out the rules for getting it right.

2.) There is one right way for sex to be. The farther one strays in thought or deed from the Traditional Model (one completely heterosexual and knowledgeable man and one woman who is slightly smaller, younger and dumber than he, united by ritual ceremony; in bed at night under the covers with the lights out, with the man on top; culminating, after a few minutes of prescribed fondling, in mutual simultaneous orgasm via penis-vagina intercourse), the less like that traditional model your predilections or practices are, the weirder that makes you, and the less likely you are to ever find happiness.

3.) There is One Right Way *you* must be in order to merit a happy relationship and sexual satisfaction. The predominant commercial norm is young, slender, fit, shiny-haired, glossy-toothed, professional, Caucasian, heterosexual, and a consumer of all the latest products. And again, the farther one is from this stereotype—middle-aged or mammoth-sized, bald, blue collar, or bisexual—the less likely you are to find love...or to deserve it.

Horsepucky, say I! If reading this book does nothing more than lessen the viselike (or perhaps *vice*-like) grip of some of these nasty notions, and encourage a compassionate chortle at the human condition we all share, it will be time well spent.

As you delve into the book which follows, I sincerely hope you will learn something which will enhance your life and your relationships with the important people in it. Equally fervently, I hope that you will enjoy yourself...and, while you're at it, enjoy someone else as well.

Bon appetít!

chapter one
A Rose by Any Other Name
(Terminology)

I've heard of engagement rings, dope rings and even faerie rings, but what on earth is a cock ring? I'd be willing to bet it doesn't have anything to do with roosters.

You're right. A cock ring is a circle of metal, or often leather, with straps that fit beneath the testicles and around the base of an erect penis. Tightly encircled in this way, the penis remains engorged at its fullest. Cock rings serve several functions. First, the wearer maintains a feeling of sexual arousal. Second, in some people's eyes, it serves as decorative jewelry, like a gold chain worn around a well-shaped ankle. Also, when worn under clothing, it "fluffs up" the genitals as in a courting display, like...er, a cock's comb. But the most popular use for a cock ring, though it doesn't work for everyone, is to restrict the flow of blood out of the engorged penis, thus prolonging erection and the uses thereof.

Maybe this is a question for a philosopher rather than a sexual Dear Abby. I'm a grown-up woman who has lived an interesting life. Is there any way you know of to distinguish between being "in love" and "in like" or "in lust"?

Like what is "attractive" or "amusing," these concepts are highly subjective, any evaluation coming from the eye (or heart, or groin) of the beholder. It will probably serve you better to try to approach each dilemma from a pragmatic standpoint— "What do I want to *do* about this unnamed feeling?"—rather than with metaphysical semantics: "What is this thing called love?" Many people have made extremely satisfactory connections, whether twenty-five-minute flirtations or years-long marriages, based on any or all of the above.

Ask Isadora

They just call it one thing in the present and something entirely different in retrospect.

You have referred to those who have undergone "gender reassignment." Since they have no reproductive capacity, these so-called male-to-female transsexuals are actually nothing more than gay male eunuchs. What they had was cosmetic surgery. They are usually eager to attract sexual attention to themselves, and for this purpose tend to conform to the stereotype of the traditional female. They wear sexually-identified rather than trade-related clothing, and practice childlike inflections rather than speak in the confident, serious tones men use. The sexual advantages of these eunuchs over real women and men are obvious: They can not get pregnant or impregnate, they have no reason to fear AIDS unless they perform oral sex on men or are intravenous drug users, and they don't even need to worry about staining the sheets one week out of every month.

My, my. I hardly know where to begin to unravel such a tangle of erroneous assumptions and faulty generalizations. First, some women who are born female are unable to conceive or bear children, and every single woman who lives long enough eventually loses the capacity to reproduce; yet we are still females, not eunuchs. While some males who undergo the experience of gender reassignment surgery are gay (men who relate sexually to other men), many are not. They related sexually to women before their operation and continue to do so afterward—as lesbians. Some were, and continue to be, bisexual. Sexual orientation (determined by whether you desire men or women) is one thing; gender (determined, at least in part, by your perception of yourself as either a man or a woman) is another thing entirely. Some transsexuals do display outdated stereotypical female behaviors; but then, so do a deplorably large number of women who do not have experimentation with new social roles as an excuse. Unfortunately, anyone who is exposed to the AIDS virus through intimate contact with contaminated body fluids can get AIDS—homosexually, heterosexually, or asexually. And finally, whatever your or your partner's gender, whenever an exciting sexual interaction takes place between the sheets, there is usually a resultant wet spot—blood, sweat, tears, whatever—on which someone has to sleep.

I'm new to the city and anxious not to appear "small town," I recently saw a piece of graffiti which I think refers to bondage games. Can you enlighten me? It said: "Dyslexics of the world, untie!"

There is such a thing as trying to be too hip for your own good. This is one of those rare instances of a joke that is not only funny, but clean, too. It refers to a reading disorder in which the reader transposes letters. My own all-time favorite bathroom exposition is: "I'm nine inches long and four inches around. Anybody interested?" Underneath, someone else has written: "Interested? I'm fascinated! How big is your dick?"

At the men's gym where I work out there is a planned body building display to show newcomers what's possible if you work hard enough. I asked a friend of mine to go see it with me. His response was, "I'm not interested in a gay T&A show." I know your love of words, Isadora. Leaving aside any political commentary on my buddy's attitude, can a man have "tits"?

Does a chicken have lips? Those bulging pectoral muscles that some body builders develop could more than fill a B-cup. But big and beautiful (and inviting to the touch) as they may be, in my mind if it's on a man it's still a chest. Appurtenances other than "pecs" which are plurals—whether tits, breasts, hooters or snow-white doves—properly belong to women. Then again, I've heard some women alleged to have "balls," so maybe it's time to broaden the interpretation of some of these sex-linked terms.

A friend of mine has just tested positive in an AIDS antibody test. What exactly does that mean and what should his next step be?

I am quoting from *The Complete Guide To Safe Sex,* authored by The Senior Faculty of The Institute For Advanced Study of Human Sexuality (Specific Press, 1987, $6.95): "Two separate tests, ELISA and Western Blot, were developed to identify antibodies to HIV (human immunodeficiency virus). The ELISA is a relatively inexpensive test, which has a higher incidence of false positives. The more accurate Western Blot is usually used to confirm a positive ELISA result. Even using both tests, a false positive or false negative result is still possible. It should be emphasized that all a positive antibody test result indicates is exposure to HIV and not that the person has or will develop AIDS." Depending on which test your friend took, his next step might well be retesting followed by information-gathering and counseling about ways to maximize his potential for a full and healthy life.

Dr. J. E. of The Haight-Ashbury Clinic in San Francisco writes: *I am a long time reader of your column and I like the advice that you give. I would like to add a bit concerning the individual with a positive HIV test. Having a positive HIV test means* more than just having been exposed to the virus, it signifies infection with the virus. This infection, unfortunately, must be considered lifelong. The person infected must also be considered infectious and has the possibility of transmitting the virus to others by sharing needles, having unsafe sex, and by donating blood, plasma, semen, or other body organs. Assuming that the individual retests positive for the HIV antibody, he or she should, at some point, meet with a doctor or nurse-practitioner and go over the medical aspects of being seropositive. This would include strategies on how to avoid stressing the immune system as well as what to look for in terms of signs and symptoms of pending immune compromise.

Thank you for your clarification. You are, or course, right.

I've always been a fan of one of the more popular satirical comic strips, which shall discreetly go unnamed, but sometimes it goes off on a tack that severely annoys me—the bit about adulterers. I know it's poking fun at sanctimonious hypocrites in public life, but I resent the inference that any coupled person who has sex outside of that couple is "cheating." I have never lied to, deceived, or cheated my wife of anything which is rightfully hers, yet I occasionally have sexual friendships which do not include her. She knows of these friendships. Would you call that cheating? Has the meaning of that word been extended to mean consenting non-monogamy?

Popular arbiters of public mores would, I think, invalidate the concept of consenting non-monogamy as a contract being entered into by person or persons not in their right mind. If you happen to be lucky enough to have an agreed-upon eating regimen which per-

Ask Isadora

mits the consumption of chocolate cake, in my book you are not "cheating" on your diet if you eat it.

I don't seem to have enough time or interest to engage in the usual forms of exercise. Can sex be considered sufficient aerobic exercise if it is done for 30–60 minutes, vigorously, about three times a week?

Most health and fitness purists would probably say not, but I've never been accused of being a purist of any sort. Since it requires no designer costumery, little in the way of equipment expense, and usually a minimum of travel to arrive at the site of the sporting event, it sounds great to me. "Go for the burn!"

Can you define premature ejaculation?

Only in my own sexual encounters. You get to define it in yours. "Premature," like "sexy" or "boring," is a highly personal judgment call. Whether we're counting in seconds, minutes or hours, if an ejaculation occurs sooner than a man or his partner would like, if its arrival is greeted with "Oops!" rather than "Ahhh" by either party, then that might be considered premature.

I've heard you mention sex toys several times. Unless you're talking about being incredibly creative with a G.I. Joe doll, a rubber ducky, or a Nerf ball, I think I'm missing something. What do you mean?

Alas, nothing incredibly creative with G.I. Joe (but if *you* think of something, let me know). Sex educators have renamed all sorts of misleading and possibly pejorative terms to reflect less judgmental attitudes. Hence, a woman who is unable to climax is *pre-orgasmic* rather than 'non'—or, worse yet, frigid. The "minor" lips of the vagina (which may well be larger in size than the "major" ones) are now more accurately called the inner lips, and the term "sex toys" has replaced the moldy old "marital aids"—which to me has always brought to mind medicinal items like trusses rather than fun-enhancers like massage oils. This new term also acknowledges that any two people can, and do, have sex, and need not be married to each other to do so.

My friend and I have an argument going on sexual semantics. When do two people actually become "lovers"? Is it once they have been sexual together or once "those words" have been uttered aloud?

It could well depend on the common usage by the people involved. A possible range of interpretations might include: "Oh yes, he was my lover. We did it in the bushes once, but I don't know his name." Or perhaps, "We've been dating for two and a half years now, but we're not lovers." This is definitely a "define-your-terms" term. Another way two people get that label, beyond the mutual decision to wear it, is through literary legend. Do people really know, or care, what precisely did or did not occur between Dante and Beatrice, David and Jonathan, Alice and Gertrude? We have reason to believe those folks did love each other, whether they said so to each other or not—therefore they have become famous as lovers, whatever they did behind closed doors.

Hey, Isadora. What is "nipple torture"? I read it in a personal ad.

It is just what it sounds like to those who wouldn't care for it. But since the nipple owner not only desires but requests such extreme stimulation as biting, clamping and pinching, I don't think "torture" is the best choice of words. "Consensual torture" is a self-cancelling phrase like "military intelligence."

I read the personal ads frequently and I notice that men wanting women who have big breasts use the term "busty." I want to write an ad to meet a man with a big penis. Any suggestions as to discreet wording?

There is a Los Angeles social group of such men and their admirers, called the Hung Jury, who put out a quarterly newsletter, *Measuring Up*. (I hear that their President "at large" is known as Taurus.) But for a local ad, there is always: "Like Stanford University" (i.e., well-endowed), though perhaps that's too discreet; "Has a big one" not enough so. Readers, I invite your solutions to this person's dilemma.

Re: the "Name That Want (But Not Too Bluntly)" Contest, here are some selected responses:

"The proper phrase is 'well hung' for a man, and, at least for me, 'well slung' for a woman."..."Full-figured male," "large physical personality," "longhorn," "man with trouser snake," "large basket," "built like Coit Tower," "virile," "big, but not chubby, guy with stamina," "want to meet a friend/lover with big...uh, hands," "doesn't go out without his Sheiks (states my preference for safe sex while it hints at size preference; Sheiks fit big penises and men who use them know that),"..."How about a bold headline of JANE SEEKS BIG DICK? (Do I get a finder's fee if she finds Mr. Big?)"..."PENIS MIGHTIER THAN THE SWORD. Female seeks well-endowed man, literary or not, to fill deep void in relationship department." Here's one ad I quote almost in its entirety:

"LOOKING FOR THE PERFECT PRINTS. I am looking for a man who can become exceptionally well-developed in a dark room, a man who by average standards would seem over-exposed in his birthday suit, a man who could call himself a tripod. Got the picture (which could fit my frame)? Please be assured that I want you for more than just your zoom lens. Photographic skills unnecessary."

One reads and hears so much about mental health. I get the sense that each "expert" has his or her own definition of it as well as a particular method of achieving it—which they'd be glad to teach you for a price. How would you define a mentally healthy person?

In her groundbreaking book *Making Contact*, family therapist Virginia Satir outlined what she called The Five Freedoms:

1.) The freedom to see and hear what is here, instead of what should be, was, or will be here.
2.) The freedom to say what one feels and thinks, instead of what one should.
3.) The freedom to feel what one feels, instead of what one ought.
4.) The freedom to ask for what one wants, instead of always waiting for permission.
5.) The freedom to take risks on one's own behalf, instead of choosing to be only "secure" and not "rocking the boat."

Given the understanding that the authority to

grant such freedoms rests within the individual who willingly pays whatever penalties may be levied for exercising them, I stand by this for as good a definition of a mentally healthy adult as any.

Recently I noticed a new product in my drugstore: Vaginal Contraceptive Film. As an amateur photographer, I am especially fascinated by the concept. Would you please tell me whether Vaginal Film is recommended for repeated exposures? Do you think it's safe for those interested in slides rather than in copies? Can it be safely used regardless of aperture size and exposure time, whether the development process is dry or wet, and whether dark rooms are mandatory?

Not to snap at you, but I do get the picture. If this clicks with my other readers, I shutter to think what may develop.

My boyfriend, whose name is Dick, avoids the obvious when referring to his genitals, but he has chosen the unfortunate alternative of calling it his Willy. There has got to be something else he can call it that won't make him squirm and make me cringe. Any suggestions?

Your question reminds me of the woman who is describing to her male dinner partner her dreams of the previous night. "Sounds pretty phallic to me," the man smirks. "Phallic?" she asks, puzzled. "Yeah, there are symbols of phalluses all through it." "Phalluses?" she asks again. In exasperation, he unzips his fly and, with a dramatic flourish, announces, "This, my dear woman, is a phallus!" Fascinated, she peers into his lap. "Oh," she finally smiles. "Like a penis...only smaller."

Anyway, one of my personal favorite names for the subject at hand is "tallywhacker." To me, it sounds neither anatomical nor threatening, but rather like something one (or two) might have fun with, like a penny whistle or a frisbee. If this isn't mutually acceptable, here are a few more: cock, dork, dong, pecker, wang (for computer buffs), wiener, skin flute, or one-eyed trouser snake.

Reader response #1: *"I read your column with great enjoyment and am especially interested in the issue of anatomic nomenclature. My British-born husband refers fondly to his "tool," which I find a pleasant and productive term. Now, what about us? "Cunt" is straightforward, historic, but frequently used as a nasty put-down. "Pussy" is kind of cute and furry-sounding, but is used as a put-down of another sort. "Mighty scabbard" perhaps, to accompany a "mighty sword"? Eighteenth century pornographers invented some flattering epithets along the lines of "honey-bedewed Temple of Venus," but that's quite a mouthful. Please ask your readers for contributions.*

Reader response #2: *Something that has bothered me for several years is that there are no power-enhancing names for women's genitals. They are either silly, cutesy, clinical, or derogatory. Can we have a contest or something?*

I, too, have been struggling for years to find something explicit, non-medical and grownup to refer, privately, to what used to be known as "down there."

Readers subsequently submitted a multitude of suggestions ranging from the poetic (*haven of pleasure*), to the prosaic (a *eunice*, for heaven's sake!). The most popular, in terms of number of times it was submitted (seven) was the Sanskrit term *yoni*. Unfortunately there's no name in this vast array that I would seriously use in conversation with my women's group, my gynecologist, or my lover. Could you, without blushing, confess to owning a *tattlemouse*? I want to tell you, however, that I am awestruck, not only by the inventive array of possibilities, but by the erudition of so many of my readers.

First, we have the tried and true: *"Since you ask for assistance, I respectfully tender the enclosed in the fond hope that my strokes of genius and the delicate touch of a linguist in this charming and sensitive area so dear to me might prove stimulating. (My god, I'm beginning to write like you!) I find* scabbard *very off-putting (and suggestive of* scab *with Freudian determinants), though I seem to recall that* vagina *is from the Latin for* sheath, *which fits nicely."*

Next: *"A big improvement over* scabbard *would be* quiver.*"* I agree, but fortunately or not, it's not applicable for all times and all occasions. Alas, sometimes it just doesn't.

"It's all very well to speak of a scabbard for the sword, but that names only the vagina and leaves out the nether lips, the mound and the field thereon, and the fiery bird nestled in the field. Perhaps one part of the problem is that the territory is more complex than the same region in men. Men have a single tool; we have a whole kit. And perhaps we could call it that. Not only is a kit *a toolkit, but also the frolicsome young of the fox. It makes sense for a foxy lady to have a kit. The Oxford English Dictionary says that a kit (workbox or basket) was originally a covered tankard. More to the point, a* kit *is also a light woman, and a small fiddle much used by dancing-masters. As a bonus, the OED gives us* kittle, *to tickle, the friction of the strings of a fiddle. Figuratively, to* kittle *is to stir with feelings of emotion, to excite, to rouse. As an adjective it means ticklish, difficult to deal with, requiring great caution or skill."*

"Here is my submission for anti-pudendal (from the Latin pudere, *to be ashamed) nomenclature:* hive, *which is grossly analogous to a*

woman's external genitalia, being hollow and subject to entering and exiting. Hives contain honey, again crudely analogous. Vaginal juices have been referred to in slang as honey. The real appropriateness of hive becomes apparent, however, when functionality is considered. A beehive is matriarchal—all bees live entirely for the pleasure of the queen, the reproductive dynamo."

That's an erudite explanation, but hardly practical in common parlance, I say.

One reader submitted a cartoon culled from the pages of *Playboy* showing an ardent male in hospital whites murmuring over a voluptuous woman spread-eagled on an examining table: "Your pudendum is like spring grass on the hills, your labia majora are the very gates to Paradise, your vagina is the infinite cosmos itself, your clitoris..."

One husband-and-wife team opted for *trouble*, as in the following exchange:

He: "I feel like getting into trouble."
She: "I have an infection. You'll
have to stay out of trouble
for a few days."

The following submission was truly an education:

"The Arabs are said to have scores of words for the female rapture aperture in all its varied shapes and moods. Till you find your own Arab informant, I suggest using the name of its possessor for the thing itself, e.g. "What does this do for your Daphne?" This literary device, in which the name of the whole is substituted for the name of the part, is called synecdoche (rhymes with Schenectady), which itself sounds like it might be another name for the subject at hand."

Ask Isadora

A Berkeley professor forwarded several scholarly articles on genital pet names from *Maledicta: The International Journal of Verbal Aggression* (Vol. 5, 1981) which suggests four categories of genital name derivations:

1.) A variation of the owner's name ("Heeeere's Daphne!").
2.) A name suggesting a joke or catch phrase (such as Wonderland for a penis called Alice).
3.) Power slang (more likely to be phallic, of course) like the "mighty sword" which started the whole thing.
4.) Human first names that appealed or occurred to the namer for no apparent reason other than it sounded right. (Where did "Dick" or "Peter" come from?)

With an international flavor:

"In England the teenagers use fanny, *which may derive from a term for a feather duster—a cone of dark feathers on a stick, suggestive of a triangle of pubic hair. This term is used otherwise in the U.S., I think. (It is, indeed.) A word one is not familiar with carries no adverse association.* Koydum *is Turkish for a really crude rendering of* cunt.

"Opak is a Serbo-Croatian word for the pointed-toe leather shoe worn by peasants. Its use implies derogatorily that the woman's vulva and vagina are old, big, worn-out and leathery." (Or, conversely, a real joy and comfort to get into, no?)

"Fustukh is Arabic for pistachio nut. It's a term of endearment, as the pussy resembles a nut and is delicious.

"Yoni—the name in the world's oldest language, Sanskrit. It's soft-sounding, exotic, and in India, actually worshipped."

Some readers revealed their own personal terminologies:

"Clish seems to be a perfect word for what it is and what it does."

"Cunty—the 'y' softens it, but also for me removes the sexual excitement of a taboo."

"Virginia—from the state's slogan: Virginia Is For Lovers."

"Tomorrow is what I call my girlfriend's because she never comes."

"Sanctuary, since it is warm, wet, and safe."

One reader opted for resurrection: *"What I would suggest is quim. It was once in robust use and carries no adverse overtones. It's grown-up, erudite even, explicit, and it is non-medical—medicinal only to the extent of its juices being a specific remedy for the ache of life."*

A traditionalist opines: *"I suppose it is clinical, but I don't find vulva too medically anatomical. However, I prefer the time-honored cunt. Every new word is going to meet the same fate as the one it replaces until attitudes change."*

Personally, I rather fancy *kit*, except for the unfortunate association that anything going anywhere near the thing would then have to be called a *kaboodle*. So, in lieu of anything better, this one gets my vote.

I'll conclude with the following poem submitted by a reader (author unknown) concerning calling Down There "it":

> The portions of a woman that appeal to
>   man's depravity
> Are constructed with considerable care,

Ask Isadora

And what at first appears to be a simple little cavity
Is in fact a most elaborate affair.
Physicians of distinction have examined these phenomena
In numerous experimental dames
They have tabulated carefully the feminine abdomina
And given them some fascinating names.
There's the vulva, the vagina, and the jolly perineum,
And the hymen, in the case of many brides,
And lots of other little things you'd like if you could see 'em,
The clitoris, and other things besides.
So isn't it a pity when we common people chatter
Of these mysteries to which I have referred,
That we use for such a delicate and complicated matter
Such a very short and ordinary word!

chapter two
The Way It's Supposed to Be
(Myths, Beliefs, and Expectations)

Ask Isadora

My husband and I are a couple of DINKS—double income, no kids. All it means is that we live a busy happy life, both of us enjoying the work we do and the interests we pursue. The problem, if it is one, is that we seldom have sex any more. It's not that either of us avoid it, or that there's any loss of warmth toward each other. It just seems like there's never any time. The fact of its absence doesn't much bother me, but the idea does, if you know what I mean. I keep thinking we should have sex X times per week or something is wrong with our marriage. Is there some frequency norm indicative of a good relationship?

There are all sorts of statistical tables showing who does what. As to their meaning, one could, if one wished, tie the number of a lover's orgasms to the rainfall in Guatemala. So what? Do you really want to run your sex life by keeping up with some mythical Joneses? If the quality and quantity of your sexual encounters is all right with you, if you are not avoiding facing an underlying difficulty by your busyness, and if you are not feeling estranged or deprived, fine. I would suggest a quiet talk with your husband about your concerns, if for no other reason than checking in: "Is this okay with you? Yes? Good, it's okay with me too." If all is well, then all is well. If not, best to work on whatever problem there is before it becomes one with a capital P. Too many people attempt to conduct their lives by what psychologist Albert Ellis calls "the tyranny of *must*urbation." You're a grown-up; you get to choose.

Isadora Alman

After careful study of the media (hunk calendars and porno flicks) and some personal research of my own, it seems to me that there is truth to the belief that black men have larger penises than white men. Do they? You're the expert.

On penises? Hardly. Some black men have larger ones than some Caucasians and Asians, yes. Beyond that I can't generalize, since penises are highly specific.

I am a 41-year-old single woman who has been sexually active since age 17. During all this time, I have never been able to have an orgasm during intercourse with any of my partners. I read an article recently that said two of the reasons for women being unable to climax are a retroverted uterus, which I have, and hormonal problems. I feel like a total failure. When I was younger it didn't bother me, but lately I'm finding that it does more and more. I have masturbated manually since I was a little girl and have always achieved delicious orgasms this way. I have had a few of my partners stimulate my clitoris manually and I did manage to orgasm; however it was not as intense as the orgasms I give myself when I do it. I enjoy sex. I don't feel I am inhibited in any way, and during the sexual act I derive great enjoyment from all aspects of intercourse, oral sex, fondling, kissing, etc. I am tired of the do-it-yourself orgasms. I want to experience the real thing with a man! Could you please tell me where I could go to seek help soon?

Suppose you were to read in this column a letter from a man whose masturbation consisted of vigorously stroking the shaft of his penis, and whose sexual activity with partners emphasized fondling and kissing his scrotum. If his complaint was that he was unable to reach climax with a partner, the problem would be obvious, right?

Ask Isadora

Somehow it isn't if the "problem" is a woman's. The lovers who stimulated you manually were closer to the mark, so to speak, but their touch wasn't exactly what you were used to, hence the less-intense orgasm. Unless you notice a change in orgasmic capacity (like being more intense right before you menstruate), the same hormones are present whether you are alone or with someone else. The angle of your uterus has little to do with it, since many women without uteruses are orgasmic.

There are several ways to look at your problem. One is to redefine it so that it isn't one: you can decide to call the pleasurable feelings you do experience with a partner "a different kind of orgasm," and thereby enjoy the events in and of themselves, perhaps bringing yourself to the familiar orgasm later as a sort of physiological "after-dinner mint." If what you want is to reach a climax in a partnered encounter, a partner can be taught to provide the kind of stimulation necessary to your achieving one—by hand, mouth, penis, or artifact. If what you want is, as you say, to reach orgasm in a particular manner (which is no more "real" than any other), then you must first teach *yourself* to respond to the kind of stimulation intercourse provides. You can learn by masturbating in new ways that include inserting something penis-like into the vagina. You can try incorporating fantasy into self and partnered sex. You can accompany intercourse with manual clitoral stimulation. (This is easier in certain positions, such as being entered from behind.)

Different sexual positions for intercourse bring pressure and friction to various genital structures like the pubic bone, vaginal entrance or "G" spot, which can produce orgasm in some women. These sensations, and the orgasms that result are likely to feel "different" from the intensity of direct clitoral stimulation—maybe better, maybe not as good as. The variety and management of the sexual responses possible for women is a topic far too vast for this space, but I do try.

With all the benefits of modern-day American life, there is one way in which our culture cripples us. We demand privacy for "personal" body functions so that learning from others as they perform natural processes is denied us. I'm 23, and I guess by now I know how to go to the bathroom properly, but I don't know how other people have sex. I suspect the porn movies I've seen are not a very accurate portrayal of what real people do. Am I right?

Yes. A commercial porn film is as far removed from a teaching device as a cartoon of *The Three Little Fishes* is from a Jacques Cousteau special. There are many sexually explicit films made for educational purposes. This does not have to mean white lab coats, charts and graphs or smarmy health professionals doing Howard Cosell imitations. The best of the educational films simply show people doing what they usually do in private. The women in them are not all young and plastic-breasted, nor do the men all possess appendages of elephantine proportions. An added bonus is that the couples who consent to be filmed for educational purposes generally are people who know and care for each other, and when that quality shows through it imbues the goings-on with an erotic charge I find sadly missing in the bawdy body flicks. It's not easy for the general public to get hold of such films, however. Try Focus International Film & Video Catalog, 14 Oregon Drive, Huntington Station, NY 11746-

Ask Isadora

2627). Also check out the sex ed classes in community colleges and universities and look for SAR (Sexual Attitude Restructuring) programs.

My lover and I are both men with lusty sexual appetites, or that's how we would have described ourselves. Lately, that's more idea than actuality. We have agreed, for obvious reasons, to not have other sexual partners; but rather than improve our sex life together, monogamy seems to have the opposite effect—nothing happenin' nowhere. Can you explain it?

Maybe. If both of you are used to a variety of sexual situations and partners, it would not be unusual if you feel angry and resentful at being deprived of them...even though you voluntarily agreed to do so. Libidos do not know from "good reasons." Talk about what is—or isn't—going on. Perhaps you can define and refine your monogamous agreement. Might it include consensual telephone sex or shared masturbation or some other safe-sex alternatives with others? If not, be creative with your lover to see whether fantasy might enhance activity. Tell each other stories, share erotic books or tapes, act out dramas complete with costumes, if that's what's called for. Your problem is not unique to gay men, but is common with many long-term exclusive couples. Each of us has many hidden facets to our personalities—the adventurer, the timid one, the child, etc. I don't care how long you've been together. It takes more than a lifetime to explore them all.

As a 45-year-old woman who has been involved for a couple of years with a man sixteen years younger, I am more than familiar with the categorical assumption that I'm in it for sex and he's in it for money. The age difference between us exists as an issue in much the same way smoking or working nights or religion exists as an issue in other relationships—something that needs adjusting to, but not something central to the basic feelings. It's worth remembering that a difference in age is not an across-the-board taboo like incest. It's more like a difference in intelligence, education, salary, height, and so on; it's fine as long as the male has more. Society seems to tolerate a gap of twenty-five years or more in the "right" direction. I think it's significant that the strongest resistance to the older woman/younger man couple usually comes from middle-aged men involved with or married to younger women.

I find it coming from men and women of any age who hate to see people succeeding by going against "the way it's supposed to be."

I am a well-educated woman who has repeatedly read that a man's penis size makes no difference in a woman's satisfaction. I guess what I'm reading is that "it shouldn't." However, it does to me. Am I wrong?

There isn't any right or wrong about feelings of sexual satisfaction. If it does for you, then it does. You feel what you feel, literally.

I am finding that the size of a man's fingers do relate to the size of his erect penis.

How nice for you. But I don't think that this is something to be counted on.

Can a person learn to be a good kisser, or is that just a natural talent some lucky people are born with?

Both. Since what constitutes a "good kisser" is a highly subjective evaluation, it's best to take specific direction from a particular kissee as to his

Ask Isadora

or her specifications. Lacking such a communicative individual, ask various members of the sex you prefer what that means to them, take the most often mentioned particulars, and generalize. At the very least, your question will lead to some lively discussions.

My boyfriend and I have been together for over five years. During this time we have become more loving, more committed and feel very close to each other. The one area that has not developed is our sexual relationship. It seems that other ways of sharing closeness have become more of a priority and we find less motivation to be sexual together. Yet we feel concerned we are not deriving the maximal potential in our relationship if we do not develop in this area. Do you have any suggestions for us?

First, have an honest heart-to-heart talk. If neither of you is actually feeling deprived, emotionally or physically, but are only plagued by some mythical standard of other people's frequency, perhaps you can let go of your "musts" and enjoy what you have. If not, embark on a course of exploration. Take a class in human sexuality at a community college, create a once-a-month Sensual Saturday Night, read some books on sexual enhancement, rent erotic videos, learn mutual massage. See what's out there that you haven't been including in your repertoire that you'd like to add, and make time for it in your lives. At the very least, all this new information will provide a few giggles, which does as much in maintenance of a loving relationship as sex does.

I had a dream the other night. In it an attractive woman, seeing that I have no erection, suggests that I take one of my mother's shoes and stick my limp zucchini into it. Then she will put her foot on top of my tool and stroke it a few times. "Trust me," she says. "This always works." Unfortunately I woke up at that point, laughing, and was unable to get my bed companion to give it a try. Would it work?

My dear, I wouldn't touch the Freudian implications of this one with a *firm* zucchini! If powdered rhinoceros horn works for some, why wouldn't Mama's old shoes work for others? They are, after all, easier to come by.

Is there a cure for premature ejaculation?

If the person whose problem this is has a partner who is also a "fast finisher" (or is a bus driver who has sex only along route stops), ejaculating quickly would be a plus rather than a problem. What you are probably talking about is that you (or your partner) ejaculates before you (or he) prefers. Learning to bring the event of ejaculation under voluntary control is very similar to toilet training—learning to recognize the symptoms before it's too late and training oneself to hold on until one reaches the appropriate place—or time. Just like with bathroom "accidents," the state of one's health and frame of mind play an important role. All things being equal, a good way to begin learning control is through practice, first by oneself—starting and stopping during masturbation, then doing the same with a cooperative partner. Eventually all the necessary signals and skills (and perhaps the participants) will come together.

I've heard that excess hair growth on the upper lip of a woman indicates a sexually passionate nature. What do you think?

How this rumor sprouted up I can't imagine. Women of dark-skinned Latin or Middle-Eastern heritage are often thought of as being

Ask Isadora

more passionate than the cooler Nordic or Anglo temperaments of blonds, and they usually have more body hair. Any connection to passion is just a lot of lip.

I am a 39-year-old woman who has lost most of my sexual desire. In my twenties and most of my thirties I had a strong sexual appetite and enjoyed it very much. Now I seldom feel like having sex, and I miss it. I keep reading that women in their 40s reach a sexual peak. Is that true? Should I seek professional help?

You haven't told me enough of your circumstances for me to even make an educated guess. Sexual appetite varies in all of us, day to day and year to year, influenced by such factors as who is in our life and how we feel about such people, how we feel about ourselves, and how we feel physically, among other things. It's not easy to feel sexual if your feet hurt, you have money worries, you don't like your mate very much, or are loath to risk yet another rejection out there in Dating Land. Take a look at your life situation. If there's no obvious clue there for why you're not feeling sexual at present, the next step is a medical checkup. A humdrum relationship or a vaginal infection is relatively easy to treat. After that, I'd start searching your psyche. The reason that women are reputed to have an upsurge of sexual interest in their forties has more to do with having finally shed some old taboos and learned more about individual wants and needs, I'm convinced, than with any sort of hormonal time clock.

For months now I've been meaning to write to you. Finally, after another four-star Saturday night and Sunday morning I take pen in hand. I am 71, my woman is 65. Neither of us was much of a performer until we met. Actually, I was over the hill. My partners—there were always two—would wait patiently for my perfunctory modest-sized heart-ons (sic) and be grateful for what they got. But (call her) Alice, by behaving like a squirming nympho, has turned me into a sensational performer. I still have difficulty getting it up, but with rampant passion I do achieve enough erection for entry when needed. Now it may be we are unique, but maybe there is an lesson here for many seniors. I think passion is the key. (Oh, I no longer need two partners.)

Not to take anything away from the uniqueness of your affair, I am reminded of Natalie and Ralph Bacon's *Love Talk* (Shakti Press, 1985), the love—and hot sex—story of the marriage of a 73-year-old impotent man and a 58-year-old former lesbian. Where there is a will, there is a way. As you have discovered, an iron erection of gargantuan proportions is no more necessary for good sex than is a variety of partners. Two people (and sometimes merely one) with enthusiasm and good will are all the ingredients necessary.

Do you think it's true that women over 45 have as much chance of finding a mate as getting hit by a flying saucer?

Not at all. But then you're reading this here. If you were reading the tabloids you might believe there was a *better* likelihood of her having a close encounter with an extraterrestrial.

Recently my lady friend flew into a rage because I declined to make love to her while she was having her menstrual period. She accused me of being a misogynist, questioned my manhood, and claimed never before to have heard of such hesitancy in a man. While it may well be that there are no health

Ask Isadora

risks associated with intercourse during menstruation, I personally find it unpleasant and messy and cannot understand how this makes me a misogynist or unmanly. More to the point, and correct me if I'm wrong, I was always under the impression that many couples take a few days off from lovemaking during this time of the month.

You are not wrong. Many cultures have enormously stringent taboos regarding what they consider "unclean" time for women. Some require them to live apart from men while they bleed. Orthodox Judaism dictates purification by ritual bathing before returning to the marriage bed. There are still myths in current mainstream society that a menstruating woman should not attempt to bake a cake since it will fall, or should not have a permanent wave put in her hair since it will fail, or that this is a completely safe period for intercourse when a woman can't get pregnant (wrong!). The only relevant truth I can offer—personal preferences, matters of esthetics and/or comfort aside—is that if a woman is infected with HIV, the AIDS-causing virus, contact with her blood can infect her partner. The danger can be diminished if he wears a condom. The messiness factor can be dealt with if she uses a diaphragm for the duration of intercourse.

Valentine's Day is a horrible time of the year for me. I'm a single woman with no Someone Special in my life except myself. That's just fine with me, but it doesn't seem to be with the rest of the world. I want neither sympathy nor other people's remedies for my situation.

My dear, you have my sympathy for your situation (no, not for your status as a single woman), but what can I do about it? Would that I could eradicate with my crusading word processor the Noah's Ark Syndrome along with a few dozen other "musts" of our screwy society. Next year, may I suggest taking to your bed between February 13th and 15th with a good book, a trusty vibrator, and some self-bought bonbons.

I am a 37-year-old male and I have not had sex with a woman (or any other living organism) since the month before my separation from my wife two years ago. I'm getting the impression from people I know who are my age, though nobody's coming right out and saying so, that a whole lot of folks are being celibate right now. I wonder how many people who are not even trying to meet people to have sex with would write to you and admit it.

I don't know what good a head count of readers, counseling clients, or even lecture audiences' sex lives would do to answer your question satisfactorily. Certainly, and appropriately, most people are being more cautious these days about sex partners. But many are not having sex because they can't, their partners won't, or there aren't any potential sex partners in their life. Whether the latter is true because they aren't looking hard enough, or at all, or are doing something—purposely or not—to turn them away, is anybody's guess. Speaking personally, two-plus years of sexual abstinence would be enough to drive me flagrantly into the marketplace. When you are psychologically ready to meet someone new or your hormones start to clamor incessantly, you'll know what to do about it.

A bus I was on recently stopped in front of a ballet poster. One lady said loudly, "Wow, is his ego inflated!" and everyone was off with comments. "It sells tickets." "I'd sure sell tickets!" "Hell, I'd show it free!" I've mentioned this to several people and they all agree that men in ballet look like their family jewels are still in the jewel box. Their crotches always seem much bigger than normal. Is there a requirement for being a ballet dancer they're not publicizing? Why not large breasts on the women to balance it out? And what do you think—can more go up than the curtain?

My grandmother, a prudish European woman of the Victorian era, said on seeing her first ballet, her attention grabbed in the same manner as the bus riders: "I wasn't aware dance was such a *manly* art." My explanation has always been that since ballet dancing in our culture has been looked down upon as "sissy" for men, wearing a protective cup under their tights which suggests enormous endowment is the dancers' form of psychological warfare: "Sissy, huh? Check this out, buddy, and weep!" (P.S. You *did* know it was a protective cup, didn't you? But that still doesn't really answer why it has to be so prominent, does it?)

As a woman of 70 retired from a rich life full of love, I would like to add a few ideas of my own to your excellent advice for women who are having trouble achieving orgasm. Often, changing the geographical location for lovemaking is the key. There is something haunting and defeating about all that hard unrewarded work in the same old bed where she's failed so many times before and even wept into her pillow. Pack up a tent to high country, book a night in a city motel, or borrow a friend's apartment while he or she sees a late movie. As for the need to feel secure before being able to relax into an orgasm, I wonder how important that is. The only two times I ever achieved deep vaginal orgasm at first sexual encounter were with men I hardly knew and never seriously expected to see again. Since I am a shy heterosexual woman, a monogamy-seeker, I recall feeling insecure on both occasions. Any illusion of security came, I think, from my distinct impression that each of these men was intent on pleasuring me first before even dreaming of having his own orgasm. With other, more secure long-term partners, I might take months to warm up to orgasm. Odd?

Not really. For many women, sex with a relative stranger frees her from any performance anxiety ("So what if he doesn't like the way I look, smell, behave, etc.—he won't be around for more than the moment!") Thus she is able to "get out of her head" and relax and enjoy herself as she would not with a man she deeply desires to impress. By the way, the tone of your letter tells me that you enjoyed the wisdom-gathering process.

I look with envy at porno films of ecstatic women getting their clits rubbed or licked. When I'm turned on my clitoris just hurts and gets irritated if it's touched directly. Then everything in me shuts down and I can't get turned on again for a while. I've had guys tell me this isn't normal and I'm beginning to feel weird. Is something anatomically wrong with me or is it that most guys don't have a soft enough touch?

Everyone has preferences about how they like to be touched, and each new sexual partner needs to be educated to your body. Consider having a medical checkup to see if you might have a chronic infection which could cause oversensitivity, but my guess is that you are the way you are and that it is normal for you. Remember, porn films are fiction, not documentaries.

Ask Isadora

I am a lesbian with an embarrassing concern: I have erotic thoughts about men. I am, and have been since my teens, a woman-identified woman for many good reasons, not only sexual attraction. I cannot imagine circumstances which would cause me to redefine myself as straight, yet what do I do with these intrusive thoughts? Should I ignore them and hope they'll go away, or explore where they might lead no matter the what consequences?

No other possibilities besides all or nothing? An individual's sexuality, as unique and convoluted as a fingerprint, can be (1.) expressed ("I desire your touch and so move my body in proximity to your hand"), (2.) suppressed ("Although I feel these feelings, you and I are strangers on the train so I will sigh regretfully and not press my haunch into your palm"), or (3.) repressed ("Sexual feelings, what sexual feelings? What I *do* have are these recurring headaches."). In the latter case it's the denial that you feel what you feel that causes psychological and/or physical problems, not denying yourself the gratification of your feelings as in the second case. (It seems a particular American phenomenon to blur that distinction.) You can decide to explore your fantasies or you can enjoy them as such without any pressing need to do anything. You can be sensual or sexual with a man without that "making you" straight. You can define yourself as woman-identified and still have a male lover or more than one.

I always figured that someone must have pinched my nipples when I was knee-high to a grasshopper and that's why I don't like to have them touched. An intimate woman friend says that in her considerable experience with straight, bi and supposedly gay men, the first group is far likelier to have this aversion than the latter two. She also says that straight men are more likely to have a tighter asshole and to be more resistant to anal insertion.

I would tend to agree, but it doesn't come with the territory biologically. All human bodies have the capacity for total body stimulation. If we define some body parts as unclean and some types of stimulation as unmanly, their erotic appeal is more likely to be denied. A man who has come to terms with who he is and what he likes, no matter how it differs from society's dictum, is far more likely to have rid himself also of such dictates: "Gee, if I'm not totally straight and I'm still okay, then it is not necessarily 'womanly' if I enjoy these sensations in my nipples either." (And, by the way, if your woman friend has had male lovers who define themselves as gay then they are not "supposedly" so.)

Occasionally, if our 4-month-old wakes when my husband and I are having sex, I bring her into our bed and nurse her. We do not exactly interrupt coitus during this time, and it is not entirely unerotic. When she has eaten and been returned to her bed we culminate our activity. Could we be damaging our child's psyche? Are we sick?

I wouldn't call you sick...sensual in the extreme, perhaps, and unfettered by customary taboos. I'm of the opinion that babies are people with all senses intact and all methods of processing information awake and functioning. She can't register your eroticism in words: "Wow, look what Mom and Dad are doing!" or necessarily remember it later in life, but I personally feel you're arousing feelings in her which are best left unassociated with family members.

Ask Isadora

Here's a follow-up:

You must not have kids. Or if you do, you must have an au pair who attends to them while you are fucking. Otherwise, you might have considered another reply to "Baby Makes Three." If you were a baby, wouldn't you rather be nursed quickly back to sleep in an atmosphere of sex-on-hold anticipation and love than be nervously nursed back to sleep by an annoyed mother glaring "Geez, give us a break already!" while your father looks on worrying that he will never be able to get hard again? As far as "registering your eroticism," do you think babies in the womb just ignore all the heat and pulsations of sex?

I have given birth, I have nursed an infant, and have I ever fucked! I am certainly not unsympathetic to the time and energy crunch of new parents. Nonetheless, I'll reiterate my stance that lust (not generalized sexuality or affection or appreciation or other warm fuzzies, but down-and-dirty high-arousal states) has no place in intrafamily, behavior and should be reserved for private moments between consenting adults.

I just started wearing makeup and wondered how to handle this. If makeup is supposed to make you look your best, then wouldn't you want to wear it in the sack? I know you're not supposed to sleep in it, but what then? Do you take it off before an amorous encounter when you're going to fall asleep afterward? Or are you supposed to slip into the bathroom to wash your face after you've made love and then wake up looking like death?

While waking up to a pale copy of the nymph one took to bed the night before is no fun, neither is resting one's head on a pillowcase besmeared with "memories." Consider wiping off "excess" (but not your complete face!) when you use the bathroom before bed. There are smudge-proof foundations and mascaras you might experiment with. Give your face a good scrubbing on those nights you sleep alone. Unless you make-up for romantic sex for an unbroken sequence of nights—in which no amount of artistry will cover your fatigue pallor—your skin probably won't suffer.

Do you ever talk about the joys of abstinence and spiritual development?
I don't know whether I would speak of its "joys" exactly, but there are certainly times in the lives of many people when abstaining from partnered sex, or masturbation, is a good and healthy choice. Abstinence as related to spiritual development, as in "conquer the animal nature to achieve higher consciousness" is not a notion I hold to at all. In fact, I avoid discussing spiritual/religious matters, along with politics. Writing about sex creates enough controversy.

chapter three
Conversations with Oneself
(Clarifying Issues)

Ask Isadora

I'm 23 and have been dating a 27-year-old attorney for one year. He's become my best friend and I love him very much. We have discussed marriage and children. However, I sometimes feel as if I have no actual animal desire for him. I remember much more passion in other relationships. Should I strike out on my own and acknowledge that maybe I'm just not attracted physically to this person? Is this a stage? Will I overcome it by spending more time and/or communicating with him? Or is desire something you can't deliver to the right person but must be instinctual? I know you haven't got a crystal ball, but I would appreciate your opinion on this.

Only in modern America has so much emphasis been put on sexual chemistry as the main criterion for making a successful marriage, and just look at our divorce statistics! Marriages have for centuries been arranged on the basis of family interests, elders' opinions of temperamental compatibility, similar life goals, and other such pragmatic concepts. Many couples who never met before their wedding day arranged a life for themselves that was satisfying, sexually and otherwise. A married life based on warm friendship and mutual respect is what many people hope for most. By all means, communicate your concerns to your friend. But only you can decide if his fine qualities are likely to suffice for a lifetime if sexual passion does not develop. If you think you might eventually feel cheated by a lack of "fireworks," think twice about marrying him and see if you can't continue a rewarding friendship while you look elsewhere for a mate.

After I've gone to bed with a man, there's always that anxious period of wondering if and when he'll want to call again. Any tips on handling that?

I'm tempted to answer that if it was good enough, he'd be a fool not to call; if he doesn't, you wouldn't want a fool like that in your life anyway. I'm afraid, however, that I'd sound more like a cross between Mr. T and Groucho Marx than the sympathetic counselor that I am. You can minimize those anxieties, but eliminating them would be like taking the fizz out of champagne. A small amount of uncertainty is a necessary ingredient of romance. You might try emphasizing in words what you have just demonstrated nonverbally—that you find his company stimulating and hope to have more of it soon. You can be the one to follow up the encounter with flowers, a note, a call, rather than sitting and fretting while you nibble your nails. You can also prequalify a sex partner to some degree by seeing beforehand if what you are looking for (an alternative to tonight's *Gilligan's Island* reruns vs. a prospective lifetime mate) is even remotely in synch with his purposes.

Is it normal to want to sleep with your father?

Freud thought so. To *do* so (sexually), however, is another matter and is against the law in all states.

I have enjoyed reading your column for some time, and I have finally summoned up the courage to write for help. I enjoy women; they make terrific sex partners. My problem is my "endowment." When fully erect, my penis is eleven inches long and quite thick. Women at work tend to go out with me because of what they have heard about me from others. I feel the women I date do so just to get a look. When they see how big I am, they

Ask Isadora

gasp and refuse penetration for fear I will hurt them. Thank god my hand is my friend. What can I do to find satisfying sex?

Very few male actors in erotic films got into that line of work because of the size of their talent. Assuming you do not want to change your area of employment, and knowing you can't change the size of your penis, all you can do is change your attitude, which helps change the attitude of others. You are what you are, you have what you have. When sexual intimacies seem likely, tell your potential partner that there might be a problem, and why. What you perceive as a problem, for many would be a fabulous solution. After the communication, use lubrication, and go about things slowly. Big events should not be rushed.

I am not sure if I am heterosexual or homosexual. I get turned on by looking at male-female contacts in books and can look at two guys going at it and get bored in a couple of seconds. I get turned on by the idea of anal stimulation, but the idea of being in a sexual relationship with a man scares me. I have talked to professional people about my doubts and they've told me I'm healthy and not to worry. I want to get a decent night's sleep. Can you tell me what to do?

For starters, many men like anal stimulation, up to and including penetration—if not by another man's penis, then by their own or a female partner's fingers, hands, or sexual toys. Secondly, sexual orientation (which sex you are attracted to) is not simply a question of either/or. There are many people who identify as bisexual, capable of being attracted to men and women, and acting on those attractions or not, for various personal reasons. Alfred Kinsey, the sexual pioneer, assigns each person interviewed in his 1950s study a number on a 0 to 6 scale, based on reported history and fantasy. (0 equals totally heterosexual in thought and deed; 6 is completely homosexual.) As with most gradient scales, only some of the subjects fall at either end. The majority fall somewhere in the middle. The professionals whom you saw obviously weren't very helpful, or you didn't stay with them long enough to get your questions answered. I strongly suggest counseling with someone who is willing and able to give you some factual information as well as explore with you your fears and fantasies.

I am a divorced woman in my 40s. To my embarrassment, I find myself having erotic dreams about my daughter's friends, young men in their late teens. What can I do about this?

Enjoy the dreams, and keep them where they are...in fantasy. Acting on them could create havoc in your relationship with your daughter. Would it be worth it?

I'm a 31-year-old gay man who has never been in what I'd call a love relationship, having always reserved that term for that special person who would come along and cause the ground under my feet to shake. About four months ago I befriended a very sweet man. Having a lot in common, we began hanging out and grew quite fond of each other. Much as I liked him, I was not sexually attracted to him since he's almost the exact opposite of my physical type—hairy where I prefer smooth, slender where I prefer muscles. However, he was very attracted to me. We did go to bed together, and while I find that we are very sensually compatible, I am still not attracted sexually. Now I feel caught. On the one hand, he

Ask Isadora

meets my psychic, spiritual, and mental needs for a partner better than almost anyone I've met. On the other hand, he is not my sexual type and doesn't hold my sexual attention. We continue to sleep together, to hold and touch, and we are very fond of each other. How do I cope with not being sexually attracted and yet feeling that this could be my lasting love?

Hot sex and soul-satisfying love do not necessarily go hand in hand (or any body part in any body part). On those rare lucky occasions when they do, they don't necessarily last for the same length of time. Lust and love have to be evaluated separately, each on its own merits, according to your own priority scale. A "lasting love" lasts because the two people involved continue to meet each other's wants and needs in some basic way. Since, in your case, your partner seems to be meeting your psychic, spiritual and mental needs, now you must decide whether the sexual chemistry might blossom later, whether you care enough about this man to call him "lover" if it does not, or whether you might construct a relationship with him that would allow for outside sexual connections when and if the ground is shaken by someone else. In any case, keep in mind that no one person can fulfill *all* our expectations. At the very least, most of us have work that is outside the love relationship, ties, and obligations to our immediate families, interests and talents that are not shared, and at least one outside confidant with whom we discuss intimate subjects (chief among them, our lover).

I am extremely happy with the man I've been seeing for some time and I am very attracted to someone at work whom I have also known for a long time, but obviously in a different capacity. Would it be pos-

sible for me to carry on a loving and sexual relationship with more than one man? Has anyone you know ever succeeded at having such multiple relationships or is it one of those idealized fantasies like "happily ever after"?

Some people have found it possible. One woman I know maintains a good marriage of more than twenty years and an additional affair with a man she has spent at least 24 hours per week with for more than seven years. Her husband also has a long-term lover in another state with whom he spends a month of each summer. Another couple I know have been together for many years in a totally open relationship. Each of them has had several affairs over the years with the new lover always being introduced to the primary partner, often becoming friends to both after the sexual affair is over. As you know, a loving and sexual one-on-one relationship takes constant tender attention and negotiations to keep both the love and the sex at optimal levels. Add the needs and wishes of another party and his or her claims on time and attention and things can get complicated indeed. So, yes, I do know that it can be done by some people. I have no idea whether you too could achieve such a "state of affairs."

I was a porn actress for a short while. The amount of pain (both emotional and physical), fear and trauma I experienced is hard to imagine. It's been over four years since I quit but I deal with it every day of my life. How do I let go of those awful memories and leave them in the past? Although my boyfriend and I are very much in love and communicate effectively, too many times I cannot separate the painful sexual memories of my past from the unrelated loving sex we share.

No amount of wishing can change the

past. Like other survivors (whether of assault, rape, or other trauma), somehow it's necessary to make your peace with what happened. Accept that it did, and accept your own part in whatever happened; and then accept yourself as you are now without guilt or blame. The key word here is not "forget," but "accept." The help of a good therapist may be invaluable here. I urge you to seek one out and lay those ghosts to rest once and for all.

I am in the military and it's been approximately four years since I have had intercourse. I have a companion, but it may be seven years before we unite. My problem with waiting so long is that I'm bothered by lust, particularly toward women of other races. This embarrasses me mightily but I thought that maybe you could be of some help. What would you do if you were in my shoes?

I can't really put myself in your shoes on the issue of being party to an agreement which would require me to go without partnered sex for up to eleven years. Is there no way your companion can be with you or visit occasionally so that you can keep the connection alive physically as well as emotionally? Would your conscience allow an open relationship—that is, relating to others in some satisfying way with the knowledge and consent of your companion? Whether your pent-up sexual feelings focus on your absent love or other women, whatever their race, there is nothing to feel embarrassed about. Those feelings are absolutely normal. (Even ex-President Jimmy Carter admitted to lusting after other women in his heart, and he was married at the time.) So your problem is not your feelings themselves, but what accommodation you can and will make to the situation you are in. Perhaps a talk with your absent love, in letter form if necessary, is the next step.

I am 27 years old and I have never had sex. I feel like a freak. What should I do?

Go about the business of living, being friendly and keeping your eyes open for potential intimates. When a friendship looks like it has the potential to become sexual, follow where it leads. You could say nothing and let nature be your guide, or disclose your inexperience at that time as an interesting piece of information about yourself. In this age of constant admonitions to check out the background of potential sexual partners, a clean slate such as yours will be regarded as a plus by many.

I am a gay person and also am religious. I am convinced that acting on my homosexual inclinations is morally wrong. I have already spent quite a bit of my limited resources looking into methods of developing and encouraging heterosexual feelings in homosexuals. The best I have been able to find was a therapist who tried to make me feel comfortable with my orientation. She said it was my religious outlook that was in need of revision! I don't believe that. What can you tell me about any newly-published ideas regarding the origin of homosexual orientation? Who might be using effective methods of making orientation changes and what are these methods? How motivated need the patient be in order for these methods to work?

For the latest books on anything to do with homosexuality I suggest browsing the shelves of specialty bookstores or a library's copy of *New Books In Print*. Unfortunately, you may think (I

Ask Isadora

think fortunately), most ethical therapists will concur with the one you saw. Just as you can wear certain clothing, affect certain stances, and develop compensating behaviors for the fact that you're short without actually growing taller, you can do the same about your homosexuality, since you see that as a shortcoming. You can sublimate your feelings for men through non-sexual friendships, marry a woman who does not expect much from you sexually, and learn to do the minimum to create a family, if that's what you want. You can make other accommodations to the fact of your homosexual urges without acting on them. But your sexual orientation—who comes to mind when you're aroused—is as "natural" to you as your height. It might be altered (in the sense of a broadened or narrowed range of responses available to you), but not changed. Anybody who promises to use some "method" on you which will make profound changes in your beliefs or your behavior is selling snake oil. Speak to your minister about low cost or no cost counseling within the ethical framework of your religious beliefs. That's what he/she is there for.

I enjoy sex very much; however, I have a problem. Whenever I get close to an orgasm the sensation becomes too much and I can't continue. If it is oral sex with my partner, I stop him. If I am masturbating, I stop myself. Why does this happen? And do you have any suggestions as to how to allow for my climax to get over that "wall"?

I don't usually encourage the use of either drugs or alcohol, but if you already use either, get a little high on your substance of choice before you next masturbate. You might also consider masturbating if you awaken in the night or before you arise in the morning and are still sleep-befogged. One of my clients (who had agreed to this beforehand) had her first orgasmic breakthrough when her lover went down on her in her sleep. What you want to do is loosen your inhibitions—sort of catch yourself unaware and with your guard down. If none of these suggestions do it, please consider seeking a sex therapist to work through whatever issues of control and surrender are getting in your way.

I am a young Hispanic woman who came to this country four years ago. I have had sexual relations three times with a boy I care about and I really enjoyed it. But since I was fourteen years old I have been having some feelings toward girls. Sometimes I feel really bad about it because I know it is against Nature. Is it a disease? Please tell me places where I can meet women like me if there are any, and what do you think—should I go?

You sound so awfully distressed about your same-sex attractions that if you acted on them now I'm afraid you might become even more upset and confused. I think it would be most helpful to you to sort out your feelings first, then decide what you want to do about them. There are many women who have sensual and/or sexual feelings for other women. Such feelings are very natural. Some choose to express them physically, others diffuse them into emotionally warm but non-physical sisterly relationships. May I suggest individual counseling first, then a woman's support and discussion group and/or events exclusively for women as a way of connecting with women on whatever basis you decide will be comfortable for you. Check newspapers for women-oriented events and the phone book's yellow pages for women's organizations.

Ask Isadora

Do you think that we still have a long way to go before there is real openness and freedom in accepting our sexuality as human beings? Another question: We are told that each woman is responsible for her own orgasm. What is your guidance in regard to female satisfaction in lovemaking?

First, who is (are?) "we"? You? Me? All of us? As a society, if some Evil Overlord wanted to drive us all crazy sexually he did a magnificent job by designing twentieth-century USA. (For starters, how about the messages woman get that there is something so terrible about their genitals that they must be kept covered, unmentioned, and deodorized, *and* they should be saved only for the man she loves: "Here, *ugh*, a present!") You must start the trek toward societal sexual freedom and openness yourself—first with yourself, then with your intimates and any children you raise. If enough people take the responsibility for educating just that small number, we'll get there. As for a woman's responsibility for her own orgasm, that's a good place to begin. It's helpful to know one's own body and communicate one's own desires. It does not mean, however, that a woman's partner is entitled to say "Well, I just got mine, Minnie, from here on in you're on your own."

I am a really jealous person, though I have been trying for a long time to get over it. Any suggestions?

Yes: keep on trying. I don't know of a more corrosive emotion. If you will take as a working hypothesis that jealousy stems from one's own feelings of inferiority (e.g., "someone will be more *this* or have better *that* than I do, and I will suffer by comparison in my lover's eyes"), you will know where to concentrate your work—perhaps with the aid of a good therapist. In the meantime, see what you can do to ease the burden on yourself. For instance, consider going to parties alone if your partner's flirting when you go together bothers you, or asking him or her to modify some particularly upsetting behavior—"It upsets me to see pinup magazines around your apartment. Would you be willing to put them discreetly away before I visit?" *not* "You must stop reading them!". The important thing to remember is that jealousy is far less often about someone else's behavior than it is about your interpretation of it.

I have been in a relationship several weeks. We laugh a lot, have a lot in common, and the chemistry is sizzling. I really am ready for and want a lifetime partner. I don't want to be disappointed for what feels like the thousandth time. How can I know for sure if this is The One?

You can't. That wisdom is granted in retrospect only at the end of your life. Now, with that disappointment under your belt, you can work on your conversations with yourself, since you are the one who keeps on disappointing you, not the men/women who repeatedly turn out not to be The One. Seize the moment. Remind yourself not that "This relationship must turn out exactly as I wish it to or it will be a failure," but that this unmapped part of a relationship is fun and exciting and scary and that wherever it leads will be an exciting adventure to be lived to its fullest.

chapter four
And All the Flesh Is Heir To
(Bodies)

Ask Isadora

This is a fairly recent and only occasional problem for me, and I am embarrassed to ask my women friends about it. Is there anything that can be done about a dry vagina?

There are many sexual lubricants on the market: K-Y, Lube, Performance. Browse in the "personal" section of a pharmacy among the tampons and suppositories or visit a sex-positive store such as Good Vibrations in San Francisco where a variety of products are available for testing. They vary as to taste, smell and viscosity. You might also take a look at whether you are aroused sufficiently on the occasions you're dry, and to what you've been taking orally. Marijuana, alcohol and certain medications all tend to dry out mucous membranes.

Is it possible to get a cerebral aneurysm from oral sex? My husband keeps pushing for it, but I'm really fearful.

Yes, and it's also possible to get hit by lightning while eating tofu alone in Muir Woods. If your real worry is medical, check with your doctor about the risk for you. But if that's an excuse for not doing what you don't want to do, be honest—with yourself and with your husband. Is cleanliness a concern? Suggest bathing together beforehand. Is it that it's unfamiliar? Read, explore, learn. If you still just don't want to, then don't. However, do explore your hesitations and give your husband the chance to see if he can meet them at least halfway. And if you do find some activity that's "halfway to oral sex," I want to hear about it.

I refer to your column on the question regarding the possibility of cerebral aneurysm resulting from oral sex. I think perhaps the woman had heard some refer-

ence to cerebral embolism rather than aneurysm. During pregnancy and the post-partum period (six weeks following childbirth), there are open veins in the lining of the uterus, and blowing into the vagina can cause air to enter these, with disastrous results. Several fatalities have been reported in the past few years. I am not aware of an air embolism being produced in this way except in conjunction with pregnancy.

Thanks for the clarification.

I'm a 30-year-old healthy male. I can always get an erection with a girlfriend, but never with a paid prostitute. Is it the lack of foreplay or is it psychological?

Both. Or neither. Or maybe some of each. In this case, your guess is a great deal better than mine. If you want to solve this puzzle without lengthy psychoanalysis, you might try two things. One, arrange time to have and receive all the foreplay you wish with your next paid companion (including taking her out to dinner) and see if that makes a difference. You might simply need to become familiar with the person whose body you are renting, a natural enough need. Two, pay attention to what your own body response might be telling you when you are about to have sex with a stranger. If you have nagging concerns about the law or catching a disease, no wonder you wilt. Your penis might be saying quite distinctly that it objects to being thrust into some strange, scary and possibly dangerous place on its own.

I'm an older woman who's been celibate for several years, and am about to remarry. A nurse-practitioner told me a year ago, "If you don't use it, you'll lose it." This sounds like a gross exaggeration and dangerous piece of advice, one that is anxiety-produc-

ing and could interfere with healthy, happy sexual relations. Would you give me some reassurances and clear up the fact from the fiction? Would vaginal fibroids interfere with enjoyment?

How long has it been since you've ridden a bicycle, and could you do so again if you tried? It's a tired old simile, but in fact, your body does retain the memory of motor patterns once learned, and will relearn them quickly. Cobwebs do not grow over unused body parts, but unexercised muscles do lose their tone and elasticity. Kegel exercises (voluntary contractions of the muscles used to control the flow of urine) and self-stimulation (masturbation) are two good ways to keep the juices flowing during long periods of celibacy. If you've undergone menopause since you were last sexually active, you may find that you don't lubricate the way you once may have, or that certain sexual positions are now uncomfortable. Since you are also concerned with growths in your vagina, gentle exploration of positions and activities with your new husband will soon allow you to accommodate your body's changes, perhaps finding new and different avenues of pleasure.

Every book I've ever read on the subject says that the size of the man's penis has no bearing on a woman's pleasure. Well, it does for me. The man I'm seeing now has many fine qualities, including being a good lover, but when we have intercourse I just don't feel "filled up." I don't see the point of telling him since there is nothing he can do about it...or is there?

The only method I know of enlarging penises (and that only works to a point, so to speak) is giving their owners loving attention. A man will only get as big as he gets. Other than finding a lover whose dimensions are more to your taste, I can suggest two kinds of sex play that will provide the feeling of a filled-up vagina. One idea is to use dildos, literally in addition to your partner. It is possible to insert a dildo vaginally and have your partner enter you at the same time, moving his penis either behind the insertion to increase length, or alongside it to increase girth. Another activity I suggest, with all due caution, is "fisting." That is, with a great deal of communication and lubrication, he can insert one, then several fingers slowly inside you until the movements usually done by a penis in a vagina are being done by his hand, open or curled into a fist. A hand with fingers is usually longer and broader than a penis, and much more nimble.

I'm a middle-aged man in my forties, healthy, divorced almost a year now. I've had a couple of chances at sex in the last few months, but my organ wouldn't cooperate with me, if you know what I mean. The whole thing was so damn embarrassing, I'm afraid to try again. So what do I do? I don't want to go without sex for the rest of my life.

To whom does your organ belong, if not to you? Part of you was not cooperating with part of you, which might very well demonstrate ambivalence—"I want to and I don't want to." First, though, have a thorough medical checkup with a doctor who is knowledgeable about sexual functioning. You may feel healthy, but failure to get an erection can be physically caused by the most unlikely things—certain drugs (both recreational and prescribed), hardening of the arteries, undetected nerve damage, or diabetes. Once you have ruled out or come to terms with a physical problem, you can look again at what you are telling yourself when you are not getting hard on demand. You might need to become comfortable with a new sexual partner first, or not continue to rely on penis-vagina sex as the main event, if you know what *I* mean.

Recently I was in Los Angeles attending the annual meeting of The American Association of Sex Educators, Counselors and Therapists. Every hour of each day offered simultaneous presentations, discussions and workshops—a veritable smorgasbord of sexual solutions. The reasons for being unable to obtain or maintain an erection are as varied as the sizes and shapes of such phenomena—attributed by various conference presenters to early childhood emotional deprivation, arterial disease, performance pressure, physical or psychological trauma, unexpressed fears or resentment, and unreal expectations. Good results in dealing with such concerns were attributed to Rational Emotive therapy, recovery from substance abuse, examining one's cultural context, penile implants, learning about sexual functions and alternative means of sexual expression, and a medically prescribed and fitted ring called The Revive System. All of these can and do work for many people. There is also a drug, papaverine, which promises what sounds like miracles. Self-injected directly into the penis, "it provides for increased arterial inflow (of blood to the genitals) which lasts for an average of two or three hours during which the male has a good erection." If ever a drug had potential for recreational abuse, this tops them all! I know little more about it other than that it has been used in erectile failure from both physical and psychological causes. Consult your friendly neighborhood urologist for more information.

My mate is considering having a vasectomy and there are a few things I'm concerned about. I know such operations are not supposed to affect sexual potency, but without sperm, won't his level of sexual desire change? Will there be any visible difference in what comes out when he comes? How soon after the operation can we safely have intercourse?

All the vasectomy does is interrupt the route from the "manufacturing plant" inside his body to the point of delivery outside his body (or inside yours). He will still manufacture sperm, but it won't go anywhere where it can have a significant effect, like fertilizing an ovum. The unexpressed sperm gets absorbed back into his body, sort of like underarm sweat from a person wearing an antiperspirant. Physically, there is no reason for sexual performance to be affected. Psychologically, some men feel less manly when they "shoot blanks." Consider that possibility from what you know of his (or your) personal notions of masculinity.

There's not likely to be a discernible difference in the ejaculate after a vasectomy. Live sperm contributes little in the way of visual subtleties, taste, consistency, or amount of liquid. Third, though some body parts may be bruised and tender immediately after the operation, sexual activity can resume whenever he feels comfortable. Since there may well be a residue of active sperm beyond the point where the vas deferens was snipped, sealed, or tied, use alternate methods of birth control until your mate takes a follow-up sperm count after about six weeks. It is a good idea to have periodic counts taken in the future as well. In a minute percentage of cases, the interrupted vas deferens rejoins itself, restoring fertility.

My girlfriend and I just moved to California. For the time being, until permanent jobs are found, we are

Ask Isadora

staying at a friend's small cottage, using the only other room besides the bedroom as our sleeping quarters. Needless to say, any sort of sexual activities are impossible. The desire, the drive, is most certainly there with her. My question is this: Is it because of this restraint put on our sex that I begin doing things to her while being sound asleep? I mean, I have absolutely no knowledge of what I'm doing until she's awake and begins doing her things to me. For both of us this is rather perplexing and slightly disturbing, although fun nonetheless.

I've heard of sleep-*walking*...! If there are going to be things that go bump in the night anyway, and you're one of those things, you might as well be awake to enjoy the encounter. There are some accommodations the two of you might make in order to have a sex life—do quieter things or quicker things (like when your host showers), come home in the afternoon, or pay for your landlord's night out at the movies. Be creative. Otherwise, since your girlfriend is co-operating, consider what's happening as a participatory wet dream, and continue to have fun.

My new boyfriend has beautiful silky blond hair. It was one of the first things I noticed about him. But his pubic hair is like a Brillo pad, and brown. Does that mean he dyes his hair, or straightens it, or what?

Maybe it's his pubic hair that's permed. Actually, there is often a big difference in the color and texture of head versus body hair. Look at beards, where you can often see astonishing variations from chin to scalp. Facial, chest, underarm and pubic hair can all vary. If the texture of his bush is bothersome, try applying creme rinse when you shower together. Even if the hair itself doesn't soften, it may seem softer in contrast to its surroundings. The process will be fun in any case.

Isadora Alman

There's an attractive man in an evening class I take. He's in a wheelchair, and since I don't see anything wrong, I guess he's paralyzed from the waist down. This isn't the only thing I'm interested in, but before I make any social openers I'd like to know whether sexual relations might be possible. Are they?

Back to the basics: sex does not always and exclusively equal penis in vagina. Since you don't identify yourself as female or male, let me also add that sex doesn't necessitate an erect penis in conjunction with any other orifice either. Sexual relations is the giving and receiving of bodily pleasure. While intercourse *per se* may not be possible with paraplegics (if this man *is* one), it sometimes is.

Even if not, that still leaves a wide variety of other body parts available and capable of offering and responding to intense, even orgasm-producing, sensations. I've heard some people say their sex life actually improved after a disabling injury or illness, since they had to learn to be creative and no longer exclusively focus on the genitals. What might be possible sexually with this particular individual requires mutual exploration, both verbal and physical, in exactly the same way the discovery of what is pleasurable takes place with any new partner who is ostensibly able-bodied.

As a male in a wheelchair, I would like to chide you slightly for your response to a letter concerning "a man in a wheelchair." I have no quarrel with your view of non-genital focusing for sexual enjoyment; indeed, advancing age underscores that. But you accepted the writer's guess that the man was paralyzed from the waist down and made a further leap that it might be due to a spinal cord injury that would make "intercourse per se often not possible." Most people—all right, we're talking about men—in

Ask Isadora

wheelchairs do not have disabilities which prevent intercourse. Polio, for example, affects muscles but does not affect genital function. Please be more careful with your assumptions and those of your correspondents.

I stand, or sit, corrected.

With everyone counseling against the exchange of bodily fluids, I'm afraid to find out for myself. I'm a gay man who wants to know what ejaculate tastes like.

Well, my dear, you have a uniquely safe opportunity to find out: taste your own. It's yours, after all; there's no exchange. May I suggest this adventure in science to all heterosexual men as well, especially those who have ever urged an unwilling female head into their laps.

The taste of ejaculate changes with body chemistry, by the way. If you've eaten scampi, it will taste of scampi. Personally, I find it tastes like watery tapioca flavored with a dash of Clorox—definitely an acquired taste.

Your revelation about the taste of semen puts a damper on a recent article on mushroom hunting. It stated that the best way to evaluate whether a wild mushroom was dangerous was to cut into it, squeeze it, and smell the resulting juice. Although written in the manner of a Boy Scout field manual, the article clearly said that if the juice smelled like human semen the fungi were probably life-threatening. As a heterosexual male whose nasal apparatus was not trained to such a sophisticated level, my solution was to telephone an escort service every time I wanted to go mushrooming. The answerer would ask for a preference and I would gee-whiz gush, "Oh, I just want her to do some mushrooming out at Land's End." The worldly procurer, not wishing to appear ignorant of some new sexual wrinkle, would never fail to reply, "Oh, mushrooming! Far out!" The gal would show up, I'd toss her a pair of L. L. Bean waders, and off we'd go. I'd pick 'em and she'd sniff 'em. Never had a problem, although it sure did make a pound's worth more expensive than buying it at Safeway. Now, according to you, semen could conceivably come in more flavors than Baskin-Robbins, reflecting what its producer ingested. Now I know the rationale for all the "hold the anchovies" orders at the pizzeria. The escort service gals were more expert than I thought, and I probably should have tipped them better.

Thank you for writing and *bon appetít*...to all concerned.

You are 100% correct when you say that what you eat affects your sex drive. If he eats a tuna salad for supper, 24 hours later a man will often get an erection. If you want an erection when you wake up in the morning, drink a glass of water about 11 p.m.

And if you *don't* want an erection try bologna (hold the mayo) while standing under a cold shower? If you believe that a tuna sandwich and tap water will do it for you then you'll be saving a lot of money on dried virgin newt or powdered rhinoceros horn. I'm delighted you think I'm right, however what I probably said was that since what you eat affects the taste and smell of your body's juices (and thus makes them either wondrous or noxious to your lovers), it will affect your sex *life*.

According to Tantra yoga, the ingestion of one's own ejaculate can have a healthy and vitalizing effect. Nutritionally speaking, would this be a way of restoring any nutrients lost during ejaculation?

I have absolutely no idea. Personally, taking

a One-A-Day vitamin pill seems a hell of a lot simpler.

On a recent television sitcom involving a character who was a male-to-female transsexual, the implication was given that the penis and testicles are cut off leaving an opening similar to or identical with an anus. I never have given much thought to the details. I'm still struck with wonder at the idea of changing sex. But surely, what the TV script implied can't be right, can it?

So much for the educational value of commercial TV. In sex reassignment surgery, the testicles inside the scrotum are the only thing actually removed. Commonly, although there are other methods, the scrotum, with its sensitivity and external hair growth, is used to form the outer lips of the new female genitalia. The penis is, in effect, turned inside out, creating a responsive vagina of a depth similar to its previous length. Nothing is done to the anus, a unisex aperture. Thinking of the female genitalia, with all their wondrous complexity, as nothing more than the absence of male genitals may have its roots in Freudian thought, but (if you'll excuse the expression) it's a piss-poor way of looking at things.

I am interested in getting circumcised. Since I don't have a regular doctor and am new to the area, I would appreciate some answers from you. First of all, how much should I expect to pay without insurance? Also, how long can I expect to wait until I am fully recovered? And, most important, is there a chance I will suffer impotence as a result of having this done as an adult?

Before responding to your letter I consulted a urologist, the medical specialist to whom an adult seeking a circumcision would be directed. The first question he asked also occurred to me: why do you want this done? Adult circumcisions are usually performed only for compelling medical reasons or as a ritual initiation. In the latter case, the head honcho of whatever tribe or religion you're seeking to join would probably instruct you as to how and by whom the rite must be performed. Since impotence is as likely to be induced psychologically as physiologically, your concerns about such a result may be very much bound to your reasons for wanting the operation in the first place. For further information about the operation, ask acquaintances to recommend a urologist or medical clinic, or look in the yellow pages of the phone book under either heading.

How do I find my G Spot, and what is it I'm looking for exactly?

The G Spot is a "zone of erogenous feeling," a highly sensitive area about the size of a coin, located a few inches inside the vagina and toward the front of the body. This particular spot was described in professional literature in 1950 by a German gynecologist, Dr. Ernst Grafenberg, and since called "G" in his honor. (I think it odd that it took so long to be written about. Over the past millennia of womankind's existence, you'd think someone might have noticed earlier—unless it appeared by spontaneous mutation.)

When this G area, rather than specific *spot*, is stimulated it produces in some women an orgasm described as deeper, more powerful, at any rate "different from" those caused by clitoral stimulation. Many women also report that stimulation of that area produces multiple orgasms, and an ejaculation of a clear fluid issuing from

Ask Isadora

the urethra which is not urine but a sort of spermless semen.

Locating it oneself is awkward. The solitary initial treasure hunt might be comfortably undertaken seated on the toilet, since pressure on that area produces the sensation of an extremely full bladder. Insert two fingers into the vagina and press up and toward the front. It's helpful if you can push down on the outside of your abdomen at the same time. (No, thank goodness, you do not have to whistle "Dixie" simultaneously!) Remember, the G Spot does not protrude like the clitoris, but it does seem to swell and harden, like the prostate, during advanced arousal stages.

If you have a helpful and curious partner, try lying face down on a bed, legs apart and hips slightly elevated. Your partner inserts two fingers, palm facing down, and with a firm touch, explores the wall of the vagina lying closest to the bed. For intercourse, this same position of rear entry, or one with the woman astride, seems to provide the most specific stimulation. If you don't find anything that feels like what I've described, don't despair. The search is half the fun.

Do you think that a widow who has not had any intercourse for three years could have a vagina that has dried up? I am 29 and my friend is a widow. The first night I had difficulty penetrating her vagina even though it was lubricated. My penis is extra large—six inches when fully erect during intercourse.

The muscles involved in the female genital system, like all other muscles, do lose tone and flexibility with disuse. You've heard the old saying, "Use it or lose it." All isn't lost, however.

Most muscle tone improves with exercise. Alas, like other muscles, the genital ones can tense up under stress, making penetration difficult. The first intercourse in three years might well be such a nervous-making occasion. I don't want to, um, prick your balloon, sir, but a six-inch erection is well within normal range, though it might be larger than that of your friend's previous partner(s). If there are more sexual encounters with this woman, take it slow and easy. You'll undoubtedly find that as she gets used to having intercourse again and to your particular body parts and rhythms things will work themselves out (or in) quite nicely.

I'm only 42, but I seem to be noticing some definite differences in my body rhythms. Could I possibly be beginning menopause at this age?

Yes. But do see a doctor. Whatever differences you're noticing could be the result of any number of things, including a hormonal imbalance.

How many positions are there for heterosexual intercourse? I've heard statements ranging from under 100 to over 1000. What's the last word?

One can count variations such as one person's head turned right, left, or thrown back as varieties of the same position, or as three different ones entirely. Multiply those possibilities by four legs, four arms, twenty fingers or forty digits—let alone the positions of items of which there are only one per couple—and you can see why interpretations on the number of positions vary so widely. Feel free to compile your own list, but like eating in all the Asian restaurants in San Francisco, while you might never reach the definitive end of such a project, the process itself is sure to be enjoyable.

Ask Isadora

I have freckles in places where very few people seem to have them. I stay out of the sun as much as possible and never go to the beach. I can sort of disguise the ones on my face with makeup and I don't wear low-cut dresses because of the ones on my chest. That's for public. But there are times in my life when I have occasion to take off my clothes in front of another person and I have sort of ended relationships before they had a real beginning because of what the other person might say. Can you help?

I can't help what another person might say about seeing your freckled nudity, but I really think you are making a big to-do over something that's more in your head than on your body. By all means, consult a dermatologist or two about the efficacy of such treatments as fading creams or even dermabrasion if you're in such great distress. But it probably would be easier to change your attitude about your freckles than it would be to alter the fact of them. Either own up to a potential partner (before the Fatal Moment) that you are very self-conscious about your coloration, so that you can hear from his or her own lips what effect it might have (my guess would be precious little), or ask for an opinion about freckles in general so you can make a *yea* or *nay* decision without personal disclosure. Again, my guess is that very few people—except people who have freckles—have any passionate feelings about them, one way or the other.

I am divorced, the mother of five. I went with a gentleman for several years and then broke up with him. While we were apart I had an affair with another man whose penis was larger. He and I had sex one day a week two or three times a day for about six weeks. I have now gone back to my old boyfriend. He says my vagina was stretched by this other man with the larger penis and this is causing him stress. I love him very much and want him to feel he doesn't need a big penis to make me happy. He satisfies me physically most of the time, but not all of the time. What can I do to make my vagina shrink back to normal? Are there exercises or special creams or lotions that will tighten this area for me? I wanted to talk to a doctor about this, but I am too embarrassed.

I suspect that the five children you bore did a lot more damage to your vaginal muscle tone than several weeks with anyone, even Gargantua, could. There are no creams, no easy solutions, but any good sexuality book will describe in detail a set of exercises which tighten and tone the pelvic floor muscles. The following is adapted from Barbach's *For Yourself*, 1975, and Crooks and Bauer's *Our Sexuality*, 2nd ed., 1973:

1. When you are urinating, stop the flow in mid-stream. You have now located the same muscles used in pelvic muscle exercises.
2. Insert a finger into the vaginal opening and contract those muscles until you can feel a squeeze.
3. Squeeze for three seconds. Relax, then repeat.
4. Squeeze and release as rapidly as possible, 10 to 25 times.
5. Imagine trying to suck something into your vagina. Hold that for three seconds.
6. Push out as during a bowel movement, only with your vagina. Hold for three seconds.
7. Three times a day do this series—exercises #3, #5, and #6 ten times each, and #4 once. These can be done anywhere, fully clothed.

You will probably notice improvement in six weeks or so.

Ask Isadora

Is it really possible for a man to be raped, and how?

The forcible penetration of any orifice (vagina, mouth, or anus) is rape. Some men can experience erections even when afraid. In those cases, even if they are technically the penetrator, it could also be considered rape. It has little to do with sex *per se,* and much to do with power abuse, exploitation, and hatred.

I am a 21-year-old woman who has been having sex for four years. All my life I have enjoyed orgasm by masturbation, and, in the past few years, through oral sex. I have always been very comfortable with my sexuality, and I am very orgasmic when clitorally stimulated. However, I have never come while having intercourse. Now I have a new boyfriend with whom I am being honest—I haven't faked orgasm as I have with many others. Is it possible for me to learn to have orgasms during intercourse, or have I become too clitorally oriented?

It isn't that you've *become* clitorally oriented, let alone too much so. That's how women are made. Our genitals are analogous to males'—the inner labia matching the material structure of the scrotum, the shaft of the clitoris the penile shaft, the clitoral hood equal to the foreskin, and the sensitive clitoral head the same as the head of the penis. How many men have you encountered who climax through scrotal friction alone? Yet that's what the prevailing myth has been for women—that a *real* woman *should* climax through intercourse. While some women do come that way, either through happy accident or through painstaking learning, the majority of women need some sort of clitoral stimulation to have an orgasm similar to the ones they've learned to recognize through masturbation.

Isadora Alman

If you want to achieve climax in any specific sexual encounter there are several ways of doing so. One is to enjoy intercourse for its own sake, receiving the clitoral stimulation you require either before or after that act—the time-honored method of "I'll do you then you do me." Another is to utilize positions where either you or your partner can stimulate your clitoris during intercourse. (I personally find this method too "busy"—sort of like a one-man band playing a tune best reserved for a piccolo solo.) Many women who do climax through intercourse alone say that it is not the same as those they achieve through clitoral stimulation—sometimes more satisfying, sometimes less so. So an alternate method is to try focusing on the specific sexual stimulation inherent in intercourse, perhaps employing fantasy at the same time. In certain positions you may find you have other sensitive spots which, when stimulated, can bring you to a "different" type of orgasm. Experiment a bit. The worst that can happen is you'll return to the tried and true with a broader knowledge of your own body and how it's best pleasured.

I am a woman who is new to having sex with other women. I am comfortable and familiar with my body, and making love with ones that are similar also feels comfortable and familiar. What's new about all this for me is how two of them fit together. I would like to come to orgasm with a partner without using fingers, hands, or external aids of any kind. Is it physically possible for two woman to find a position so that their clitorises touch?

Where there is a will, there is (almost always) a way. Half the fun of being with any new partner, let alone one of a new gender, is experimentation. Many woman find ways to receive the stimulation necessary for their orgasm by lying face to face or one astride the other and moving so that friction or pressure on the pubic bone and areas around the external sex organs is sufficient. A position which would at least bring the labial areas into close approximation is a scissors-like arrangement of legs with heads at different ends of the bed. If your partner is not knowledgeable enough to suggest something once you say what you want to achieve, look through the well-illustrated *Joys of Lesbian Sex* (Sisly and Harris, Wallaby Books, $12.95) for something that looks like it might work for you. If you are unable to find such a position after the search for it has ceased to be fun, consider relaxing your requirements that orgasm must occur in any particular way. They all feel good.

When my penis contracts during ejaculation and orgasm, it feels as if my anus is contracting at the same time. Does it?

Are you really asking *me* if *yours* does? A simple way to find out is to reach down, or back, when the moment approaches and feel for yourself. Most people's do.

I am a woman with a burning question: since I am prone to hemorrhoids, should I avoid anal sex? The few times I've tried it, it caused a sharp pain. My boyfriend tells me it just takes a little relaxation and I'm willing to try—if my hemorrhoids aren't bothering me. Will anal penetration irritate them? A gay male friend of mine says that anal sex is actually good for hemorrhoids. Can he be right?

I have also heard that anal sex is good for hemorrhoids, but I've never spoken to a living person who was willing to try that as a remedy while he or she was having a hemorrhoidal flare-up. Several factors are to be considered here. The anus loosens and relaxes with heightened arousal, as does the vagina; like the vagina, it also tightens up to repel entry when its owner feels threatened. Pain is not a necessary accompaniment to anal sex, but it's a definite cease-and-desist signal, whether you've got hemorrhoids or not. Since the anus produces no lubrication of its own, use lots—on you and on your boyfriend's penis or whatever is doing the penetrating. The best time I know of to attempt anal penetration is just before or after you climax. You are likely to be either so wildly excited you forget your fear, or so relaxed and happy there is none. Go slowly; when it ceases to feel good, stop. Try again some other way or some other time. The guidelines for anal sex in general are: "Lots of communication, lots of lubrication." And at the risk of sounding like your mother, don't forget your rubbers. Unprotected anal sex is definitely not a safe practice.

I've always had one breast smaller than the other, but in the last year I've realized they are now the same size. Can the growth of one breast be attributed to frequent sex over the last two years?

I doubt it. It's normal to have a discrepancy in size on most matching body parts (breasts, hands, feet, testicles). Your breast increase *could* be due to overall weight gain, muscular development, constantly doing something vigorous with the hand and arm on that side, or a late growth spurt, but I'd certainly have yourself checked out by a doctor.

My boyfriend's erect penis is nothing to sneeze at, being of average or better length and girth. At rest, however, the shaft virtually disappears. He

Ask Isadora

looks like he has an acorn between his legs. If I had met him first at a nudist colony I might not have furthered the acquaintance, if you know what I mean. Is there any way to estimate penis size for a clothed man, or erection size for a penis at rest?

What comes to mind is "Ya pays yer money and ya takes yer chances," an ancient punchline of some now-forgotten vaudeville routine. No, there is not much correlation between penis size soft and hard. Short ones just get proportionally larger (more than doubling in size from two inches to five inches versus an increase of 25% from four inches to five inches, for example). If one at rest dangles six or more inches you can be fairly sure that it won't *shrink* as it hardens, but beware of assumptions. There was a porno actor who hung at some preposterous length like ten or eleven inches, but who didn't seem to ever get hard. It's my belief that if enough blood flowed into that appendage to harden it, the poor guy would faint from lack of oxygen to the brain! As for estimating erection size of a clothed man...one of the most awesomely proportioned I've ever, um, come across was on a man less than 5' 5" tall and one of the smallest on a six-footer. Who says Nature doesn't have a sense of humor?

Every time my girlfriend has an orgasm she expels up to a cup of what appears to be water from her vagina. This is not the normal vaginal lubrication that occurs during arousal. She is 28, healthy, and has experienced this since she's been sexually active. We would like to know what's happening here. How common is it? Should one try to control it? Any tips on cleaning up the excess liquid would be greatly appreciated.

There is a possibility that if sex usually occurs right after she has taken a bath, gone swimming, used a douche, or the like, that she is expelling, by the orgasmic contractions of her vaginal canal, water which remained trapped therein. What is more likely is that your girlfriend is a member of the minority of women, exact number unknown, who ejaculate. The liquid you (and others who have experience with this phenomenon) describe is watery—not viscous like lubrication, not acidic like urine—and seems to be expelled from the urethra. The news that there are women who do ejaculate and exactly what they ejaculate is still controversial. An attempt to control this fluid gush by women who thought they were urinating, for example, often results in an inhibited orgasm. Add a large towel or plastic sheet to whatever else usually accompanies your bedtime fun, and enjoy the fact that you're sharing the responsibility for creating the wet spot that no one likes to sleep in.

I have just read in your column about a female who expels about a cup of fluid during orgasm. I would like to add my two bits (or two cups). I, too, come like crazy during peak periods of sexual activity. And, yes, it is just the consistency and nature you describe. It has caused me a certain amount of embarrassment and insecurity, especially with a new or inexperienced partner. However, at 35, I've grown accustomed to my sexuality and consider myself lucky to possess such a tangible sign of my excitement and openness. I am only curious to know more about how "minor" the number of women is who do ejaculate.

I know of no statistics, but I do keep "abreast" of new research, and am happy to keep you posted. I am not asking anyone else to stand up, towel in hand, to be publicly counted, but I am one of the juicy minority. Since I don't remember experiencing this phenomenon until after I turned 40, there may be some advantages to ageing not yet tallied. (If you are one of my former lovers who feels moved to write in and dispute me, reminding me that another advantage of advancing years is an erratic memory, please restrain yourself.)

Thank you for suggesting that some of the rest of us "stand up, towel in hand, to be counted." I never ejaculated before my 39th birthday and it has happened fairly regularly into my forties. Dr. Dean Edell, in a memorable news column, said "females cannot ejaculate; they have no semen," and then went on to say that in fact, the fluid was urine. I was never so offended in my life. The fluid I expel is nothing like urine and it doesn't come from the bladder, but rather splashes off the vaginal walls. My partners have been easily able to discern that no urinating was going on here. Poor Dr. Edell has clearly had no personal experience with this phenomenon.

Okay, honey, do you get to educate him or do I?

When I was younger I would ejaculate when arousal was strong. Later on, nothing, even though I was married to the same man, though less sexually aroused by him. Maybe the phenomenon has something to do with the depth of arousal.

Ladas, Whipple and Perry, the folks who wrote *The G Spot*, feel that stimulation of this area on the upper front vaginal wall is what is likely to produce female ejaculation. Ejaculating at some points in your life and not at others may also have to do with physical changes in the vagina itself, perhaps through age and/or childbirth. I think as you do that the intensity of the turn-on is as much of a factor as the method.

There are certain things my partner and I do sexually which I find quite painful. What can I do about this?

"Add more lubrication" is a response which covers a goodly percentage of the things I can think of that you might be doing, but without more specifics I'm really at a loss. What comes to mind is that old vaudeville routine: "Doctor, it hurts when I do this." "That's easy to cure; don't do that."

My new girlfriend and I get along extremely well, and sex too has been very good. There is, of course a problem, or else I wouldn't be writing to you. I don't like going down on her because she has an extremely pungent aroma—very acid, and overpoweringly strong. Cleanliness is not the issue. She showers every day and sometimes twice. It's just that the minute her juices start flowing—and they do that considerably—the strong scent appears. What can be done about this and, since she seems unaware of any problem, how do I tell her that there is one from my point of view?

The same way porcupines make love—verrrry carefully. "You smell bad" is never a heart-warming message, and I think "You taste bad" would be worse. You are dealing, in more ways than one, with a very sensitive area—her feminine essence. You could not mention any problem and just work around it, so to speak, either by never going down on her, or doing so only briefly until she gets musky, or only on specific occasions, such as in the shower or right after a bath. You know I espouse the cause of honest communications, but that does not imply the

Ask Isadora

necessity of telling your partner everything always. If there really is nothing she can do about it (change her diet, douche with parsley juice, think of baseball scores while you're doing her so that she doesn't get turned on), then why cause discomfort for both of you? —Which you undoubtedly will by bringing it up.

You sure dropped the ball when the guy asked how he should deal with his lady's disagreeable vaginal odor. This last year my own partner broached the subject with me. His understanding and educated example is worth publicizing. First off he asked, "Are you under a lot of stress these days?" Pause for answer. "Well my nose is close to the natural perfumes of your body right here, and your body changes odor all the time. Lately it's terribly pungent, and I'm concerned." He previously told me he knew when my period was coming, that it has a sweet smell. We discussed tension, dietary change, physical checkups and good health. He told me he has encountered this phenomenon with other partners. I still don't know why it happens, but if I suspect it, I do a light douche with bicarbonate of soda. I don't want to be deprived of a crucial part of my sexual pleasure. Who else can tell me but my lover? We have a good thing going and he cares. So if that guy had enough passion and care to write to you, you should have provided him with better guidance.

Maybe he could take her into one of those exotic sex shops, and along with a couple of new sex toys to experiment with, pick up a few flavored love potions, especially a flavored douche. If I was her I would be more than willing to try all sorts of things to make oral sex better for my lover, for to simply forego it, as you suggested, would be a great loss for me.

Onward.

Isadora Alman

My boyfriend's foreskin covers his entire glans, despite his claiming that he was circumcised at birth. Is this possible? Can you give me an estimate of the cost of having this foreskin removed? I would like to give him this surgery for his next birthday.

Talk about what to give the man who has everything! What would you bestow on the next occasion—a nose job? I have never heard of a foreskin growing back after it has been removed. I might guess that the original circumcision (if indeed one was done and not some other procedure) was performed incompletely or inadequately. Whatever the case, giving someone surprise elective surgery is not my idea of a tactful gift. If the presence of his foreskin bothers your boyfriend as much as it does you, perhaps together you might visit a urologist to discuss the situation. If not, ask him to wear an opaque condom and proceed as usual.

Six years ago, after having a complete hysterectomy at age 37, my body hair began to disappear. I am divorced, and this is so embarrassing to me that I have avoided sexual encounters rather than explain this to a new man. My gynecologist has no explanation for me. I've taken estrogen and progesterone for the past three years, but it hasn't made any difference. Can you help me?

I can't help you grow hair, but perhaps an endocrinologist (someone who specializes in disorders of body chemistry) can shed light on the matter. I suppose it wouldn't help to remind you how many many women spend many many dollars on depilatories, razors, waxing salons, etc. to achieve the lack of hair you deplore. (Nah. I didn't think it would.) There truly exists an object called a merkin, a feminine pubic hairpiece. However, in my opinion it would be far more profitable for you to work on changing your attitude about your lack of body hair than on the fact itself. I have no doubt that there are as many, if not more, men who would find body baldness a turn-on than a turn-off; and my guess is that the majority of people wouldn't give the whole business a second thought. When you approach the stage of a relationship where baring your all seems imminent, confess your misgivings, listen to what your partner says about it, believe him, and go and enjoy yourself.

A few years ago I met a man and fell in love with him, and he with me. When I first became aware of him in a romantic manner, strange things started happening to my body—things I had never felt before for anyone. My ears would itch, then my lips, and then my bottom. After a while these reactions stopped. But now, since we broke up three months ago, they have started all over again. What are these reactions to him that don't stop even though we are not together any more?

Itching is often a nervous reaction. You might have felt nervous about falling in love initially, and nervousness about the recent breakup. Because you never felt like this before it is not to be taken as some cosmic sign of special affection—"This must be Mr. Right! I feel it in my skin!" This could also be something as prosaic as body lice you caught from him and are now left with, or an allergic reaction to something entirely apart from him. If it doesn't go away, consider seeing a dermatologist first, a psychotherapist second.

I have four questions on the same topic: 1. Are there many women out there who prefer uncircumcised penises and why? 2. Is it a myth that uncircumcised ones don't get as fully erect? 3. If it's not needed, why are men born with a foreskin at all? 4. Is adult circumcision common?

1. Yes (although, as I've said often enough, few women accept or reject a potential lover solely on that basis); and I don't know why—a matter of what you're used to, I suppose, anteaters or rockets.

2. Yes, it is a myth except in certain problem cases, which can be surgically corrected.

3. I don't know. If you speak to the Designer about it, ask about the appendix while you're at it.

4. As I mentioned earlier on, adult circumcision is usually performed only for compelling medical reasons or in cases of conversion to a religion that requires it. Medical and popular opinion are leaning more and more toward abandoning the practice, that, in this country, has been almost automatic at birth for years.

I've had little luck in eroticizing latex and the bottom line seems to be the amount of sensation I feel. Like the great majority of American males my age (40s), I am circumcised...with the inevitable decrease in sensitivity. Wearing a condom over my already desensitized penis makes it feel even more wooden. Isn't the practice of routine circumcision setting the country up for the AIDS epidemic since it decreases sensation and thereby increases the resistance to using condoms?

Had I been born the lithe and lovely daughter of royalty I am sure my life experiences would be different, possibly richer, than they have been; but since I was not, how can I ever know? If you are not one of the relatively small number of men circumcised after sexual maturity you can only imagine a compared loss of sensitivity as I can about my life as a ravishing princess. If you have strong ideological feelings on the matter, by all means, become politically active in the campaigns to abolish routine circumcision. But blaming your distaste for condoms, let alone the AIDS epidemic, on circumcision is illogical. Most men do just fine with their "desensitized" members, among them those eager ejaculators who would be delighted with a little less exquisite sensitivity. Encourage safe erotic touching that de-emphasizes or replaces intercourse, experiment with condom brands until you find the thinnest possible, add lubricant to the inside to increase your sensation, and only as a very last resort would I consider a foreskin restoration.

I am a young woman with a very embarrassing problem. For the past three years when I have an orgasm I lose control of my bowels and bladder. It's gotten so bad that I only dare masturbate on the toilet. Forget about partners. I have asked two doctors about this but they have both avoided the question. I am miserable. Where can I turn?

An immediate solution is to prepare for a sexual encounter by restricting food and liquid intake for several hours ahead of time and taking an enema directly before. Since most doctors have pathetically little sex education, they tend to be just as uncomfortable with the topic as the rest of humanity. Ask for recommendations for a gynecologist and/or proctologist from friends or your other health care providers. Call the office of that physician and tell the receptionist you have a sexual problem and would like to speak briefly to the doctor on the phone to know if it is within the doctor's area of specialization. A few minutes of conversation should tell you if you've found someone willing and able to deal with your concern.

Isadora Alman

I am a healthy man in my 30s. Since I split up with my wife a while back I've had a few short relationships, but in each one I've been more or less impotent. It seems that this problem has been the reason none of these women wanted to stick around. I didn't have this problem with my wife and I don't have it when I'm alone. I've been in psychotherapy since the split but I don't seem to be getting any closer to resolving this. I feel like what I need is a woman who is loose, understanding and a little patient too, but there don't seem to be too many of these around. AIDS has killed the sex surrogate approach and I don't want to mess with prostitutes. Any suggestions?

Yes. Ask your therapist for a referral to someone who specializes in sexuality. If you are happy with your present progress in other areas there need not be a conflict; the two could work with each other and with you. That adjunct therapist could well be a sexual surrogate. All the members of IPSA (International Professional Surrogates Association, P.O. Box 74156, Los Angeles 90004) check their health thoroughly and often, use safe sex techniques, and, depending on what they might be doing together, often require a medical checkup on their clients as well. While there might be many women willing to be loving and patient while you face this challenge, I don't think you can expect that kind of attention in a brand-new relationship, at least not until a bond of trust and affection has been formed on both sides. But by all means, continue social outreach as well, and perhaps you'll get lucky.

Settle an argument please. Doesn't the presence of testosterone in men account for their higher sex drive?

Ask Isadora

Amounts of testosterone vary within and among men *and* women. The amount at any given time may be one of the reasons many men often want sex more than many women, but always? I state with certainty that there are no absolutes. Some women often want more sex than many men do!

Does a man lose zinc through ejaculation? If he ejaculates often (say 3 times a day) will he have a zinc deficiency? Can this deficiency be made up for by ingesting zinc supplements?

It's extremely rare that a body will *deplete* a natural substance through a natural process. (If you excrete a lot through sweating, for example, you will feel thirsty to compensate for water loss.) Ejaculation in any quantity the body is capable of will not in itself cause a zinc deficiency. If any exists, it's probably due to diet or pathology. A nutritionist is the person to consult, first, to establish if a deficiency exists, and second, about rectifying it.

My man gives hot head in more ways than one. This may be a dumb question, but when a man eats hot chiles and then goes down on you, can it irritate that delicate tissue?

Sí. So...olé!

chapter five
Fantasy and Friction
(Solo Sex)

Ask Isadora

I frequently enjoy using a vibrator during masturbation to bring me to orgasm. However, a friend tells me that excessive (whatever that is) use of a vibrator will make me dependent upon it, gradually dulling my response to partner sex and diminishing my capacity to reach orgasm during "normal" sex. Tell me it isn't true!

Orgasms achieved through vibrators are often more intense than those gotten from other sources because the stimulation is more reliable than the customary human partner is capable of providing. And some people do get hooked on high-intensity sensations. One hopes, however, that partnered sex offers compensatory benefits—affection, conversation, even a theater companion, which not even the most advanced mechanism is yet capable of providing. It is also to be hoped that the pleasure in, and appetite for, such peripherals will keep your libido turned outward occasionally. If no satisfactory orgasm results from a particular partnered interaction, you can use that trusty recourse sitting in your bedside drawer and get all the above-mentioned goodies without performance pressure. Isn't that the best of both worlds?

I'm a married woman, and my relations—including the sexual ones—with my husband are fine. Occasionally he works late, and I find I look forward to those evenings alone. Sometimes I take the time to masturbate, and often I don't feel right about that. Do you think I'm cheating him?

Did you give him exclusive rights to all of your orgasms when you married him? They are yours to create and/or dispense as you choose. Self-pleasuring is exactly that, and marital lovemaking distinctly something else. It isn't a matter of either/or but of both/and. You might consider discussing the subject with your husband if it will set your mind at ease—not in order to get his permission, but in the spirit of clearing the air of guilty secrets or sharing intimate disclosures. If the fact that you enjoy an occasional evening by yourself intensifies your guilt, look at the commuter traffic on any given morning and notice the preponderance of single-occupant cars. For many people, that's the only time they are ever alone, and they guard that opportunity jealously in the face of all commonsense reasons to carpool. Even for the most devoted of couples, time alone and apart is necessary to replenish both the partners and the relationship. I find a lot of truth in old blues song titles. One of my favorites is "How Can I Miss You If You Won't Go Away?"

I read your column with wide-open eyes, learning something new each time. I am a 68-year-old woman without what you so nicely call "a partner." I'm a widow. I never knew women could pleasure themselves sexually. How does one go about that?

There are some very good books on the subject—Lonnie Barbach's *For Yourself* and Betty Dodson's *Sex For One* are two classics. Some therapists run pre-orgasmic women's groups with no age limit whatsoever. You might call San Francisco Sex Information (415/621-7300) and ask a volunteer to share her practices and methods with you. But even never having attempted it, in this case you are the expert, or soon will be. May I suggest a luxurious bath, a bottle of non-perfumed body lotion, good music, and setting aside an hour or so for sensual exploration. When you happen upon a body part that feels especially good when stroked, continue. When you "shift gears" in the sexual response cycle from sensual pleasure to sexual excitement,

Ask Isadora

you'll know the feeling and almost automatically continue the stimulation that feels right to you. If you feel uneasy about touching your own genitals, use directed sprays of warm water (such as those from a handheld shower nozzle) or use a hand-size massager to the same effect. Allow your mind to wander to whatever romantic or erotic images appear, or choose one and tell yourself a bedtime story. Remember, the aim of this is your pleasure, not performance. If you don't reach a climax the first few times, I hope the experience will be delightful enough to encourage repeated experiments.

I am a 20-year-old male. My problem: I am a chronic masturbator. I know it's natural for people to masturbate, and I have no worries about growing hair on my palms or anything, but I do feel my masturbating is excessive. I've been in situations where I'd rather not stop to answer the phone! This may not sound serious to you, but I sometimes feel that I have masturbated my life away, and I worry that it will affect my performance with others. I wonder if there's anyone else out there with the same problem.

You are not alone. There are times when I, too, would rather not stop what I'm doing to answer the phone, and I'm not doing anything half as entertaining. You are right, though, that frequent masturbation, if done with the intent of reaching climax as quickly and as often as possible, may well affect your performance with a partner. If, when you do it, you concentrate on prolonging the process, finding new and surprising ways to enhance the pleasure of the journey without hurrying toward its destination, and accompany the event with fantasies about meeting potential lovers and the delightful things you will do to and with them, you may find that you want to get out there and actualize those fantasies. In this way you can pleasure yourself and, at the same time, motivate yourself to do something other than remain at home ignoring the phone. You might then become a sensual and imaginative sexual partner and, when the happy coupling occurs, feel that rather than having wasted the first twenty years of your life, you were using them well for warm-up and conditioning.

I babysit a little girl who is just about one year old. Like a lot of kids, she has a favorite stuffed animal she likes to sleep with. When I put her down for a nap, instead of cuddling Teddy in her arms, she lies on top of him (which can't be comfortable) and sort of humps on him with her pelvis. If I try to move the toy, she gets upset. If I leave her alone with it, she humps it until her face gets red and she stiffens and quivers all over. I can't think of any other explanation than that she's masturbating to orgasm. Is that possible at her age?

Yes, and from what you describe, very probable. Orgasm is a time-honored natural method of releasing body tension before sleep. Allow her to enjoy herself. There will be time enough for her to learn the socialization rules of our culture. When she begins to play with other children, she'll find out that some pleasurable activities, like picking one's nose, are best reserved for private time.

It turns me on to watch my friend masturbate. Is that all right?

Is it all right to be turned on by watching someone else behaving sexually? Sure, that's the whole basis for the erotic film and video industry. So your response is certainly within the realm

Ask Isadora

of "normal" behavior—if that's what you're asking. It is *not* all right to involve another person in your sex life (with the exception of solitary fantasies) without his or her consent. If your friend knows you're watching, it's probably a turn on to her or him that you do. If your friend does not know, and what you are doing is "peeping," it's not only rude and dishonest (unless cleared in advance), in many circumstances it's also against the law.

I have masturbated frequently over the past ten years. My "habit" began at a time when I was not having sex. I now lead a normal and active sexual life, but I lapse into masturbation "spells" even during relationships. I occasionally do this using pornography even though I feel uncomfortable with it in the house. Can the pornographic images I project cause unforeseen distortions of reality? Am I doing any potential harm to my body? Your comments would be appreciated.

Masturbation *is* a part of a normal sex life. In most statistical surveys more than 60% of women and 90% of men report doing it. It's no more a substitute for another kind of sex than salad is a substitute for spaghetti. You might have a preference for one or the other sometimes or settle for second choice on the occasions your first is not easily available, but a well-balanced diet includes both. As for the pornographic images—that's not as clear-cut an issue. If the fantasy images you hold get in the way of your relating to real people, causing disappointment that his penis is not twelve inches long and spouting like a geyser, for instance, or requiring any woman to have missile-shaped breasts and a staple in her navel in order to be deemed a turn-on, then it is distorting reality. In the end, your own ethics and personal politics have to be the deciding factors on what you deem acceptable erotica vs. pornographic trash which demeans both you and others.

On the radio I heard you respond to a woman who expressed concern about the fact that her partner sometimes masturbated several times a day. Even without a complete description of the man's behavior, I think some mention of the emerging theories of sex and love addiction would benefit this couple and anyone who hears you. Based on the 12 step program of Alcoholics Anonymous, Love and Sex Addicts Anonymous offers supportive group meetings for those of us whose sexual or romantic fantasies and actions have come to dominate our lives. I don't mean to imply that this is necessarily the case with the man who masturbated frequently, but compulsive sexual behavior or a habitual need to be romantically involved can be as addictive and hard to quit as drugs. Deception and justification can only work so long. Eventually it becomes all too clear that one's productive life has taken second place to the obsession. There are many people for whom sex or love has become a regular escape which results in more pain than pleasure.

I agree that many people feel stuck repeating behavior which no longer serves them. Changing a habit, particular one which has in the past reduced tension, is really difficult. Any help in doing so, especially from people who have been there, as in the AA model, is a good deed indeed. I personally have a great deal of trouble, though, with the term "addiction" when we are not talking about a substance but a behavior. Call it compulsive behavior if you must. I don't much like that term either, but we are all in agreement that whatever behavior we are discussing is involuntary (as in against one's own better judgment), whether it's saying "um," overspending, or flashing in the park. In the case you refer to, it would be up to the man who masturbates and not his partner to decide if what he was doing was "too much," "a bad habit," or resulting in more pain than pleasure for *him*.

I've been using a vibrator to reach orgasm for a long time. I've recently switched to manual stimulation and the orgasms are not as intense. Will they get more so if I continue to use manual stimulation, or is this as good as it gets?

Unlike Gertrude Stein's rose, and regardless of what Masters and Johnson's instruments show, an orgasm is not an orgasm is not an orgasm. The location of the stimulation, its duration and intensity, your feelings about the stimulator and even the phases of the moon all enter into your perceived satisfaction with the orgasm it may induce. Very few human beings can keep up the intense and unvarying stimulation of a vibrator no matter what body part they use (although I have had fantasies about bluegrass banjo strummers). So if "intense" is your criterion of good, you may want to stick mainly to your handy appliance.

chapter six
The Opposite Sex
(Men/Women)

Ask Isadora

I know that it's my responsibility to see that I have an orgasm if I want one with a partner, but as a woman, how do I control a man's ejaculation?

Oh, my dear, men have a difficult enough time with that issue on their end, so to speak. Briefly though, if you learn what movements, pressure, position and words are most likely to trigger an ejaculation for a particular man, do them when you want to induce one and refrain from those particular things when you hope to delay it. Good luck.

There is something I have been wondering about. Is multiple orgasm a strictly psychological phenomenon for women?

For some, yes; but that doesn't make the feelings any less real. For some women it's strictly physical—keep providing the correct stimulus and you'll keep getting the expected response. Very Pavlovian. For many women it's a combination of several factors—the right setting, person, activity, mood, etc. The same is true for men, by the way. Men are capable of multiple orgasms, though generally not multiple ejaculations. We're talking about a peak sensation (from pretty damn nice to heavenly bliss) followed by feelings of peace and completion, however short-lived.

Do most men enjoy oral sex? As a woman, being on the receiving end is my favorite activity.

I doubt if I can give you a generic answer. It's true that being the recipient of oral sex is many women's preferred, if not only, route to orgasm. Different men feel different ways about doing it, from enthusiastic to repelled. Let your man know your wishes and hope fervently that he's one of those who fall on the better end of the scale, or has potential of becoming one. Since there's some ambiguity in your question, let me add that receiving oral sex is not a universal delight to all men either. When it comes to sexual preferences, there is never an absolute.

Is it true that women get turned on by men's bottoms?

Some do, some don't, and some can be distracted by intelligence, wit, and other less "fundamental" characteristics.

When Halloween comes around every would-be drag queen comes tottering out of his closet wearing all the stuff that shouldn't be in there. I'm a man, and I dress like one 365 days a year. Don't real women feel outraged when they see all those insulting caricatures? I would.

I'm a real woman, second in that department to no one except the late Mae West, and I love playing dress-up. I only feel uncomfortable when some guy pulls off in jest what I've been working on for never-mind-how-many years...and does it better! As I often say, being a man has little to do with having a stiff prick. The same applies to being one.

I've recently signed up with a dating service. I filled out a questionnaire about my likes and dislikes and they sent me a list of profiles of women they selected. I have no idea if their criterion is anything more than those who have signed up for their service. All the women on the list they sent me are 35 or older. That's okay with me, but how does a woman feel about dating a younger man? I'm 32.

Which woman? Your question seems to expect an all-purpose generalization like "Women always..." or "Women never..." There aren't any of those in my repertoire. Contact the women on the list who seem most promising and make sure that among the other tidbits of information you offer or they ask (like education, job, interests, etc.) you volunteer your age as well. If she consents to meet with you, the air has been cleared on that particular issue and you can go on to more important considerations such as whether you enjoy each other's company.

In a previous column you wrote about gender reassignment. I have difficulty untangling your convoluted thinking. Even though I am a psychiatrist, I'm unable to figure out any rational motivation for a man who is heterosexual and who "related sexually to women before his operation" having his penis cut off in order to appear to be a woman and to ostensibly function in that role. Other than homosexuality, which you feel is not necessarily the case, what motivation would you attribute to such behavior?

The clients you see in your practice, Doctor, must differ vastly from the ones I see in mine if you require behavior that is inexplicable to you to stem from "rational motivation." The motivation I might attribute to anyone's behavior is beside the point until I understand theirs. The person who wants all his teeth pulled out to stop the Martians from broadcasting messages through his fillings has a good reason to do so from his own point of view, if not from yours, mine, or his dentist's. Therefore I asked a woman friend of mine (who was born with male genitals) to respond to your letter:

"A rational reason for a heterosexual man to have a sex change to enable him to relate sexually with women as a 'pretend female'? In a single word—none. A 'man' would not change his genitals for anybody or anything. A woman-identified person would, if the genitals bothered her enough. Men who pale at the idea of cutting off their genitals obviously are male in body, mind and spirit. Men who have their genitals cut off for whatever reason are indeed most likely to be extremely unhappy, or at least, so I suspect. On the other hand, a person who perceives herself as having the sexual identity of a woman and who has the misfortune of having been born with male instead of female genitals might welcome the opportunity to reshape them to match her sexual identity. She ought to be deliriously happy with this solution, regardless of her sexual preference. Even as a lesbian, I certainly am...and so are my lovers. By the way, if the person asking the question is implying that surgically altered genitals can't be just as sexually satisfying (if not more so) than the original unwanted ones, then he is sadly mistaken. At any rate, I urge him to hang on to his with both hands."

You answered a letter from two men in a long-term relationship whose lack of sexual desire for each other was bothering them. I am a woman of 41, my female partner is 38. We've been together for seven years. There's lots of holding and hugging, warmth and wonder in our relationship, but as for hot sex...? I can't really remember the last time. It has to be years. I think if that fact troubled my lover she'd say something about it. It doesn't bother me. I'm not writing about any problem then, I guess. Just wondering whether, in your experience, you find this a men versus women phenomenon, or just a matter of individual differences.

Both. On a statistical average men's libidos are more insistent than women's. Analogously, men are taller than women. But we all know that there are many men under 5'6", and many women taller than that. The man who wrote me described himself and his lover as "men with lusty sexual appetites," so it was the departure from *their* personal norm which was disturbing. When the desire for sex—whether frequent, nonexistent, or somewhere in between—is relatively equal between two people in an intimate relationship, there is usually no problem, as in your case. When it is perceived as a problem anyway, as with the male writer, the dissatisfaction is due to measuring sexual frequency against some other standard like "what we used to have" or "what other couples report having." While a reduction in the frequency of sex affects most long-term couples, it does seem to be extremely common in female couples. Women are theoretically more "relationship-oriented," valuing affection over sex, and are the traditional responders rather than initiators. If no one initiates sex, what is there to respond to? Whether that's due more to the difference in the nature of women or their acculturation, I don't know. I think it's a combination of factors.

I'm a successful woman with a full life, but an empty bra. I'm seriously considering a breast augmentation. How important are big boobs in defining "sexually attractive" to men?

To some men—very; to others—not at all. To still others—sometimes it is and sometimes it isn't. During your lifetime, you're likely to encounter a few of each persuasion. How you feel about yourself as a sexually attractive woman is the most important question.

I have noticed a lot of women who wear tight pants, which I enjoy, but I am puzzled by one thing. Some of the women wear their pants so tight that their sexual organs are outlined perfectly. They might as well wear no pants. Do they realize this? If they do, do they get their kicks this way?

Probably; and some might.

A couple of weeks ago I heard a caller on your radio show who described himself as a 42-year-old male virgin. The pain in his voice was poignant. It sounded as if you've encountered this problem before.

Several "late bloomers" have consulted with me. The problem is not as rare as you might think although its definition varies widely, with some people still pondering their future entrance into the awesome world of sexuality well into their forties and fifties, and others in their early twenties sure that they'll never catch up because they are still inexperienced.

As a longtime reader of the personal ads, there is one noticeable and repetitive theme that I, as an older woman, find particularly disturbing—older men and their desires for younger women. Today, women are living longer, taking better care of their bodies and mental health, and have sexual cravings longer, but their chances for partners in their own age group are sadly diminished with seven women to every man over 50. It appears that 85% of the males who place personal ads indicate their desire for women 12 to 15 years their junior. What is it that younger women have that mature, healthy, interesting, educated, playful, enthusiastic women in that man's peer group do not? Are these men afraid to confront their physical counterparts with the gray hairs, wrinkles and sagging skin that we all undergo as we age? I sense that maybe a need for status plays a part in their search for a youthful partner to reassure themselves that they are sexually okay. I have found that men ten to fifteen years older than I have not been able to keep up sexually, neither with their energy level nor

Ask Isadora

with their erections. My feeling is that it doesn't matter to me as a mature, experienced woman. I can get gratification just from knowing that someone is interested in me as something more than a sexual object. Let's hope you can generate some honest response and clarification on this situation. I personally feel very put down and out by this ageist attitude.

Me too. If I believed that *all* men wanted the wish list of young, slim, smokeless sexiness I see perpetually advertised for, I'd resign myself to knitting alone in my rocking chair. Fortunately, I don't believe it for an instant because my rocking chair is currently being repaired...it broke under the strain of sexual excess my much younger lover and I put it through.

Reader response: Regarding the woman who wrote complaining that there are seven women to every man over 50: Her discussion of gray hair, wrinkles, and sagging skin is, I suspect, talked about in the bedroom. I can almost hear her: "I'm aware that I don't look so good, and I understand that you are older and that your energy is flagging, and that you're unable to get an erection like a younger man. It doesn't matter to me as a mature, experienced woman." And then she wonders why he does not call her again! She requested some honest response and clarification. I think that the primary problem is not the faulty statistics she quotes (her 7 to 1 ratio is way off), but rather her complaining in the bedroom. As for me, I run away from the scorekeepers of any age. Happily, there are women out there who appreciate gentle, slow lovemaking which has been nurtured and developed by experience and, yes, partially as a result of age.

I think what this woman was asking was if there are any *men* out there who also appreciate those qualities.

My husband passed away ten months ago. I am 48 and haven't had sexual intercourse until just this month. With my new man I reach climax during intercourse when I am on top. Do other women use this intercourse position?

Yes.

A woman recently said to me, "Men act as if they are doing a woman a big favor by taking her out." I feel that many women act as if they are doing me a big favor by accepting my offer of a date. I am a divorced man in my late 50s, and while some women I've been dating are glad to accept my dates, they never phone me. If I don't phone them again and invite them, I'll never see them or hear from them again. I feel I don't matter much to them, and that doesn't feel good.

Many women of your generation (and mine) simply don't feel it's proper to ask for or initiate *anything*—whether it's conversation or sex—and need some encouragement. Sweetly and clearly tell your women friends what you want. If you make it a statement of your preference ("I feel valued when a woman phones to invite me somewhere, even to a walk in the park"), rather than a demand, ("If you want to see me again it's your turn to call"), you will receive pertinent information. If she answers "Oh, I couldn't call a man," tell her what you've just told me. If she hears you, says nothing, and still doesn't call, you can then turn your attentions toward a more productive relationship—one wherein the woman is pleased to please you and where the question of who is doing whom a favor simply doesn't arise.

I am 51 and have been divorced twice. During my periods of singleness I've dated perhaps 100 men.

Ask Isadora

It seems typical of men, particularly widowers or men just out of long-term relationships, to assume that they can pick up with a new woman where they left off with the last one and to compare you unfavorably with their ex. What many a man seems to overlook is that the last woman he was with was his wife. He made a commitment to her. She must have felt secure with him and did not wonder if she was ever going to see him again, probably did not wonder if he was doing the same thing with someone(s) else, was reasonably sure they would be spending Christmas and New Year's Eve together, and that he cared about her welfare. Yet this same man expects the same kind of unrestrained sexual enthusiasm from a woman to whom he's made no commitment and has known relatively briefly with little attempt at courtship, romance, tenderness, or even a hint of a future date! I believe that in most cases it takes a long time to develop a really trusting, satisfying, and exhilarating relationship. These guys want an instant replacement without going through the necessary steps.

Most people who are hungry will recall fondly the last food they bolted down. No matter how dry and unappetizing it really was, from their current perspective it becomes a feast. I think you—and most probably the men you speak of—are confusing expectations with hope and fantasy. Most ex-spouses/lovers were not instantly responsive multi-orgasmic marvels. We must not tar—or feather—all men with the same brush. You may have dated a run of sex-starved men, not at all a rare commodity. Simply explain to any prospective lover who seems to be rushing things that for you it takes time to develop the trust to become sexually responsive. That's true of most people, by the way, not just you or women in general. And while most people are aware of that fact, and concur, to some the prospect of even mediocre sex looks infinitely better than none at all.

How can I find out what turns a woman on?
Ah, the old "what do women want?" dilemma. For a good general overview, any library or book store will have a selection of books on female sexuality. If some activity shows up again and again in women's reports or fantasies, it's probably a pretty safe bet that many—though not all—women will respond to it, whatever it is. With a specific woman, either ask, experiment, or try an interesting melange of the two.

I have always envied women their ability to have orgasm after orgasm. Is that natural to them (maybe to offset Nature's dirty trick of having to bleed every month), or is it acquired learning?
Just because the books say women are capable of multiple orgasm does not mean that *all* women are, or even that all women want to be. Some come naturally (so to speak) to that phenomenon, others seem to develop the ability as they grow older (perhaps another of Nature's compensations). For some, one orgasm is grand, glorious and sufficient. In my experience, a very short recovery period between orgasms, or what looks like none, is more likely with climaxes reached by other than clitoral stimulation. Ongoing direct orgasm-producing stimulation of the clitoris with a tongue or a vibrator often numbs a women out sooner that it tires her out.

Is it pretty common for a woman to need something more than intercourse in order to reach orgasm?
Yes.

I grew up in modest circumstances, but at the

age of 31 I've achieved more than I ever dreamed I would. The most striking change brought on by success is the way I'm treated by women. Suddenly I'm six-feet-four and have looks that rival Redford's! I hope I won't be blamed for a simple observation, but after a lifetime of watching women's behavior, both from the sidelines and now as a "winner," it seems to me that women are ready to sell themselves to the highest bidder, expecting a property interest in a man's future. They offer sexual access in return. If that's what women are offering, some men would prefer to keep it on a per-transaction basis. As for me, I really don't want it that badly.

Robert Redford himself has said in interviews that until he became a star women were scarce in his life. So even looks that *are* Redford's don't always help. There is nothing new in the fact that some women consider money and success the ultimate aphrodisiac. And some women are whores and some men are johns. Long may their unions prosper. They deserve each other. As for you, your "simple observation" about the nature of all women will turn into self-fulfilling prophecy unless you acquire some new social circles as well as some badly-needed attitude adjustment.

chapter seven
Without Unwanted Consequences
(Sexually Transmitted Conditions)

Ask Isadora

I haven't dated in a long time and am just starting to get back into the swing of things, so I have a few crucial questions. Should I take an AIDS test so I will be able to present myself as safe to my new suitors? If so, does one need to retake the test every few months? If you "pass" the test, are there still reasons you could be considered unsafe? And how unsafe is doing oral sex on a man?

Let me see if I can give you the basics here. AIDS is just one of several possible diseases transmissable through unprotected intercourse. You can become infected with the virus which causes it in any single encounter with the blood or semen of an infected partner; therefore, every unprotected sexual encounter which includes intercourse is a possible occasion for transmission of anything from the HIV virus to the common cold. What's being tested for is not AIDS but the presence of antibodies to the virus which may take the body as long as six months to produce (i.e. only showing up as a "positive" test result six months after infection). Obviously then, a test every few months just won't do it. Your best bet is to only engage in practices which do not put you at risk. (Safer-sex guidelines are available from the National AIDS Hotline: 800/342-7514) In performing oral sex, avoid mouth contact with either semen or the clear secretions some men produce during arousal.

I've been getting a weekly massage at my health club for several years. I think the guy who gives the massages might be gay. Am I in danger of catching anything from that contact?

If you've been seeing this guy for years and still don't know his sexual proclivities, then you haven't had the kind of contact likely to endanger you. Relax and enjoy.

Isadora Alman

I'm from Houston and I come to San Francisco three months out of the year for jobs in the area. I so greatly want to be faithful to my loving wife that to satisfy my sexual needs when I'm here I go to porno booths and masturbate. I go just about every night. I'm so fearful, though, that I can catch AIDS or some other disease. Could you please shed some light on this for me?

To catch a sexually transmitted disease of any kind, *direct intimate* contact with another's body fluid is required. I know those booths are not as clean as Mom's kitchen floor, but if you watch what you sit on or rub against you should remain perfectly safe.

Whenever you and other sex educators discuss oral "safe sex," condoms and products with Nonoxynol-9 are mentioned, as if fellatio is all that's involved. When cunnilingus is mentioned, what is and is not safe sex turns unclear. Is it because transmission from female to male performing cunnilingus is impossible? Unlikely?

Honestly, I don't know. The AIDS virus has been cultured from all the body fluids of an infected person, with the highest concentration found in blood and semen. But it's also there in sweat, saliva, tears, and vaginal secretions. Whether in dangerous amounts or not is just not known. If you are a female loath to forgo the pleasures of being stimulated in this way, your best reassurance to a partner is a certified clean bill of health. Second best: a latex square called a dental dam available through supply houses or via your dentist. That's not saying there will therefore be *no* risk, but it may lean those undecided in your favor. And man or woman, the one who comes up with something like a condom for the tongue will be hailed as a hero by many.

Ask Isadora

There are no cases of female-to-female transmission of AIDS. I checked with the San Francisco AIDS information number and with the Center For Disease Control, which is the national authority on AIDS statistics. The AIDS virus has been around for more than ten years, and not a single case has been attributed to saliva, sweat, or tears. Why not urge your readers to pick up the phone and call the CDC (404/329-3286)?

While the CDC is the recognized authority on AIDS statistics, what they disseminate can be weeks in the gathering and open to various interpretations. New information, or at least theories, about AIDS transmission, hit the daily media often months before publication in medical journals. My own information about *possible* female-to-female transmission comes from a discussion with a member of The AWARE Project, a UCSF study. What we know now is not the last word about AIDS incubation and transmission patterns. It's all too new. I have no wish to be a fear-monger, but isn't it better to be safe than sorry? Who wants to be dead right?

I am a 23-year-old male college student with a few questions about AIDS. One, can I be exposed to the AIDS virus while receiving oral sex, since the only ejaculate involved is my own? Two, when a guy ejaculates on his partner's chest, is there any danger when it lands there, broken skin or not, or is the virus killed when it's exposed to air?

We are getting into areas of risk assessment here that can only be dealt with in degrees of "likely" or "unlikely." Certainly the recipient of fellatio is at much less risk than the one who receives the semen. If the fellator carries the AIDS virus it will appear in his/her saliva, but *probably* in insignificant amounts. The broken skin issue, whether on penis, chest, or other body parts seems iffy too. Are we talking about a pimple or an open bleeding wound? The situations you describe seem relatively safe for you.

A very attractive man I met recently seemed to shut off any further possibilities between us by informing me that he had recently tested positive on the AIDS antibody test. Can you explain clearly what that means? Is he necessarily a "carrier"? Am I crazy to contemplate any kind of relationship with him?

A positive result means that the individual in question has the virus in his system. A full health examination in the face of that information is always advisable, not only to rule out the possibility of error, but to learn about taking precautions against coming down with any of the several diseases which now validate a diagnosis of AIDS. Meanwhile, as long as you avoid contact with his blood or semen (as well as saliva if you want to feel super-safe) you can form any kind of relationship at all with him, assuming he's willing. Understand that in the first shock at the news of his test result, he may feel appallingly vulnerable and you may have to be fairly direct and persuasive to get things moving. Perhaps reviewing safe sex techniques together may reassure him that an HIV positive diagnosis need not mean that his sex life, affectional life, and indeed, his very life itself, is over.

Recently at a cheap peep show and at a gay porno movie house I witnessed unrestrained group sex acts with guys going at it like drowning people grabbing at straws. No one was washing between or after each act. One guy had visible open sores on his body. (I'm 60 years old and 50 pounds overweight and I had to beat them off.) I phoned one of the AIDS hotlines and was told by a bitchy young man that I was acting like an old fart trying to spoil their fun and if I didn't like what was going on, just not to go back. What can I do?

You can toss condoms and safe sex pamphlets into such melees like a modern Johnny Appleseed, or you can report such goings-on to either the Health Department or local police who have the power to shut down such establishments if flagrant health violations are occurring. What you can't do is change certain people's "hell-bent for death" attitude about random anonymous sex. Your feelings are not that of an "old fart" or party-pooper, but a concerned human being. Think about putting your outrage-induced energy to good use and consider becoming involved in some community-wide health education projects.

The issues of safety and trust have come up for me recently because my boyfriend is starting to see other people. Is there any such thing as a safe sex instructor, someone a person can go to in order to learn new techniques?

Any up-to-date sex educator or knowledgeable counselor is essentially a safe sex instructor. You could schedule a private counseling session or two in order to deal with your specific questions. Such counselors teach sexual techniques through films, books, dialogue, etc. If it's "hands on" teaching you refer to, that's the province of sex surrogates. Referral to work with a surrogate, male or female according to your orientation, is just one of the resources in the repertoire of a good sex counselor. Counseling is an educational tool. One doesn't need to be sick or broken in order to use it for maximum benefit.

Isadora Alman

Here's a hypothetical situation: Two young guys fall in love. They are both virgins. Neither have had recent transfusions or are intravenous drug users. They maintain a monogamous relationship. Assuming they are aware of safe sex practices such as condom use, must oral sex be avoided? Do they face the same high risk of AIDS as people who have had active sex lives?

Virgins and people with long sex histories do not face the same risks. Being gay in and of itself is not a risk factor, nor is contact with healthy semen. If you are as you've described above and you are asking me to asses your risk of catching or transmitting AIDS, I'd call it extremely unlikely.

I fear the AIDS problem is being exploited by erotophobes and moralists who wish to return to more sexually repressed times. It would be a shame for hard-won sexual freedoms to be lost due to a scare that has little basis in fact. Please comment on the real risks the average sexually active heterosexual faces in contracting this deadly disease

There is no research that I as a sex educator am privy to which is denied to you. Regardless of the hysteria of some doomsayers or the denial of whistlers in the dark, AIDS can strike many "unlikely" people—newborns, a celibate who may have had a years-ago blood transfusion for dental surgery, the monogamous spouse of an infected person. I base my behavior on my judicious interpretation of all that I hear and read; you must do the same.

I am appalled at how few "low risk" people test themselves for AIDS. Besides people who donate blood regularly and some responsible gays and bisexuals, no one else seems to be doing it. Since I person-

Ask Isadora

ally don't know a single person who uses condoms regularly (including me), my feeling is that condom use will never be widespread enough to have an effective impact on stopping the spread of disease. With testing, however, I think far fewer people would be exposing their lovers to AIDS if they knew they had the antibodies. You are in a position to reach so many responsible sexual people. Please encourage people to get tested voluntarily.

I certainly share your concern, but I cannot in good conscience encourage willy-nilly test taking. Although there are steps to be taken to prolong good health if the results indicate HIV infection, such a result is not remediable the way some other venereal disease might be. Unless one feels capable of handling the outcome of testing, whatever it is, I think it's better to assume you or anyone could be infectious and take precautions as a matter of course. Not using condoms yourself but relying on the honesty of unknown partners who report having been tested is foolhardy in the extreme.

I have had a primary sexual relationship with my wife for several years. Recently, I have become involved with another woman who has several sex partners. My wife and I are concerned about the risk of AIDS. How great is our risk compared to high-risk groups? Is "safe sex" our only option in loving each other and others responsibly?

I'm afraid so. Since you can't know the history or practices of your partner's other partners, "high-risk groups" may be closer to home than you think. These days, "they" are "us".

I'm a recently-divorced man in my 40s, who's looking forward to many new sexual experiences, none of which is having herpes. Is it true that a cer-

tain percentage of adults can't get herpes because they already have the antibodies?

We all know stories of people who "never" get poison oak or are "apparently" sterile and wind up with nasty surprises. Herpes is a virus—a group of several viruses, actually—and who is susceptible when is still unknown. All I can tell you for sure is that some commonsense precautions on your part are...well, just common sense. If you make it a rule to always use condoms for any sort of intromission, even when preventing pregnancy is not an issue, contracting or passing on herpes will be one less worry. While having herpes is not the end of the world, nor of a sexual life, if it is possible to avoid exposure, do.

I have had periodic cold sores on the corner of my mouth since I was a child. That's not the same as herpes, is it?

That's exactly what it is. If your reaction to that statement is one of horror or doom, do you see why some people believe that ignorance is bliss? Herpes, whether oral or genital, is not necessarily a sexually transmitted disease (you need not have contracted it that way originally), but it is spread by physical contact. If you refrain from kissing, sharing cigarettes or face towels, and other common health measures during your outbreaks, you need not feel any more of a social pariah now that you know than you did when you believed that what you had was "only" a cold sore.

I was diagnosed as having trichomonas and informed my (only) partner of eight months. I thought it was the adult thing to do; I knew it was inevitable that he would give it to another woman. He told me he had no symptoms and a urinalysis

Ask Isadora

proved he was "clean." Various health professionals told me that men are 95% asymptomatic, but can infect their partners, causing a "ping-pong effect." Unless he plans to be celibate for the rest of his life—fat chance!—he's going to cause problems. What do you think of a man who refuses to be treated for trichomonas?

As you know, even a man who tests "clean" can still be a carrier of trichomonas. Those little critters are hard to spot. I can understand his reluctance to undertake a program of strong medication to cure a condition he neither suffers from, nor ever apparently has. I can also understand your indignation at the possibility of being re-infected, or of his uncaringly infecting someone else. The preferred treatment for this condition is to medicate both people in an ongoing couple to avoid the ping-pong reinfection of each other which you mentioned. But if he refuses to be treated, I know of no way of *making* him. To protect yourself, you might insist he use a condom during any future sexual intercourse between you. As for protecting other women, short of taking out a personal ad—"Beware! Ira Irresponsible carries cooties!"—I can't suggest a thing. It is possible to contract trichomonas nonsexually, so be aware of slander and libel laws.

I've taken to heart all the admonishments on safe sex and want to do my part. I'm embarrassed to admit that as a man of 33 I've never bought a condom, let alone put one on. Who do I ask for advice on such an intimate matter?

Isadora, of course. Most urban drugstore chains have condoms on open display. No need to shout your order to a pharmacist who looks like your mother. There is a bewildering array of prices, types, and, though the packaging won't

Isadora Alman

say so for obvious reasons, sizes. If you can't find a sampler package of a variety of styles, buy several singles or three-packs to try at home. Some major distinctions are: pre-lubricated or not, entirely form-fitting or with a little reservoir tip on the end to collect the ejaculate, smooth exteriors or lumps and bumps (theoretically designed for the recipient's pleasure), and made from latex or animal intestine. The old days when the invariable thickness of these products made the wearing of them comparable to taking a shower in a raincoat are fortunately over. Some condoms have in their lubrication an additive called Nonoxynol-9, a preventive of some sexually transmissible diseases. Do experiment with several brands to find your optimal fit. To put them on, you or your partner should apply the folded circle to the end of a penis which is at least partially erect and roll it on gently over the shaft as far as will go. Whatever the style of the condom's tip, always leave a bit of room at the end to catch the ejaculate and to accommodate a larger erection.

A word or two about linear lovemaking—that is, following a pattern of some of this and that leading to intercourse, with ejaculation as the grand finale. Simply stated, it doesn't have to be that way. If the condom wearer loses his erection, just check that the condom stays relatively in place, or remove it and put on another if (re)insertion is imminent. You and your partner should be the ones to dictate the course of your sexual activities. Condoms do not yet have the vote. Be sure to hold on to the top edge of the condom when withdrawing from vagina or anus, otherwise you might leave it inside unwittingly. In this case, you not only *can* take it with you, you must.

Ask Isadora

I've found at least one way to handle the unpleasant taste of semen. My man and I experimented with condoms for birth control a few months back, buying three to the pack and trying them for fit, feel, etc. The results are that the thinner and tighter they fit the penis, the better they feel to both of us. I like the non-reservoir type the best. It's also best to lubricate the head of his penis before putting it on. I wondered how they tasted and tried them for this too because I really like to feel the contractions when he comes in my mouth. They didn't taste nearly as bad as I first imagined. (I also discovered that if you are in a hot 69 some men don't even know when you put one on them.)

I trust that you purchase the type of condoms that are externally unlubricated? As for putting a condom on an unwitting partner—do be sure to take it off as well, or he might be in for quite a surprise when he stumbles into a dark bathroom to urinate afterward.

I am a 35-year-old man who is no stranger to either sex or human anatomy. Birth control has never been an issue for me because I am sterile from a childhood illness. (Yes, I've been tested.) With things being the way they are these days, I purchased a pack of well-advertised, general-price-range condoms to accustom myself to their use. I was appalled to discover that they were too large, or at least they certainly didn't fit like the "second skin" I'd expected. I thought they were one-size-fits-all. I know I'm not that substandard or someone, including me, would have noticed. What gives? Any explanation?

All condoms are not the same size. Manufacturers are not likely to label them Small, Medium and Large for obvious reasons, but I don't see why they can't be sized like laundry detergents where the smallest one available is called Giant. The way things are now, one simply has to experiment to find not only the desirable features but comfortable fit as well. Certain types are best for thick penises rather than thin, curved rather than straight, and, yes, large ones rather than...not as large. Some sex shops sell variety packs of condoms, and I've seen them in mail order catalogs, but for some reason I haven't seen any in pharmacies.

The Institute for Advanced Study of Human Sexuality has assembled a Personal Safe Sex Sampler Kit which is for sale through them, all proceeds going to research on AIDS and general sexual health education. The reason I mention it is that in the description of the package contents a Hugger brand condom is followed in parentheses by the word "small," which is the first time I've ever seen such helpful information in print. (The condom packet itself says "made to fit snugger," which is ambiguous.) An anonymous message on my office answering machine recommended Man-To-Man condoms as running large. This is a brand which the above mentioned Institute evaluates positively in their booklet, *Safe Sex In The Age Of AIDS*, but they make no mention of whether it is wider, longer, or stretchier than average.

When I was a kid, Trojan was used generically for "rubber"; but when I tried the standard regular Trojans they were so loose they affected both safety and self-confidence. My father, a very buttoned-up man, told me the following story when I was a teenager: One prostitute asks another how her business is going. "Oh," she replies, "same old sixes and sevens." (The American Heritage Dictionary defines the slang term as "in a state of disorder or confusion.") Without intending to, I'm sure, my dad

Ask Isadora

allayed my penis size anxiety once and for all. So here's another recommendation for your condom list: Conceptrol Shields. I've found them easy to put on, yet snug enough to help prolong pre- and post-ejaculation performance. While I'm on the subject of size, I'll share another adolescent discovery: It was fun to play with the cardboard core from a toilet paper roll, which fit me in the same snug way.

Thank you for your suggestions. Cardboard rolls sound like a far more ecologically sound, not to mention ethically correct, sex toy than the family pet.

My problem is that my boyfriend refuses to buy or use condoms. I think I've come up with a solution. What if I put rubbing alcohol on his penis before sex? Would that make it germ-free and sanitized?

It might work for a door knob, but not a man's. Even if your boyfriend were willing to stand (or lie) still for your ministrations, you yourself would have a very rude surprise when the alcohol on him came into contact with your own tender parts. I hate to be the one to discourage creative thinking, honey, but this time it's back to the drawing board, or better yet, the negotiating table.

What's a guy to do when his condom won't stay on? I've tried them all but my foreskin invariably "shimmies" them off. Do other uncircumcised men have this problem? Short of belated circumcision, which I'm frankly unwilling to have done in any event, what might you suggest?

Experiment with rubber "O" rings available where plumbing supplies are sold. See if you can find one tight enough to hold the condom in place and loose enough to do it comfortably. A friend of mine anchors his condoms by enfolding a few pubic hairs in the fully unrolled condom then rolling the lip back over again once or twice. If the condom begins to slide, the tiny tugs on the attached hairs are the best of attention grabbers. If that idea sounds only slightly more appealing than adult circumcision, try Mentors, a condom brand which contains an adhesive to keep it in place on the penis shaft.

I am a gay man, and for oral sex I use Gold Circle condoms because they don't have that numbing rubber taste. Since these are non-lubricated, I also use a lubricant inside, but there is a problem. After ejaculation I sting when I urinate—very badly and painfully. Is it the Nonoxynol reacting with the rubber, do you think? I use condoms with the same lubricant for non-oral sex and I don't have this problem, even though they too are rubber or latex. Do you know another condom which doesn't have a taste and might be used? Help me solve this burning question.

Both Ramses and Trojan make lube-free condoms, but I don't think that's the problem. The massaging action of your partner's tongue during oral sex might be pushing the lube up into the urinary passage and what you experience afterward is a mild allergic reaction to the Nonoxynol-9. What I'd try is a lubricant without it for masturbation and receiving oral sex only, reserving that with the added protection for contacts of greater risk.

I am a gay man. I don't know about the circles other people travel in, but my friends customarily say hello and goodbye with a kiss on the mouth. The kiss itself can range from a t.v. talk show purse-lipped kind of smack to a deep soul kiss. At least three people I see socially have been diagnosed AIDS antibody

Ask Isadora

positive, yet their lips and tongues are right in there with the rest of them. I know you are extremely unlikely to pass along the AIDS virus from saliva, still.... What do you think about all this social kissy-face in this day and age?

I would be offended if any person but my very nearest and extremely dearest stuck a tongue in my mouth on any occasion, let alone as a casual social gesture. Leaving aside for the moment the state of either party's health, non-mutual tongue thrusting is downright rude. (If one is not well, it's abominably thoughtless.) The way you can indicate non-consent without being rude in return is by presenting a cheek to be kissed, offering a warm embrace which bypasses mouths, or turn aside a kiss by saying, "Forgive me, I don't want to pass along my cold."

Once and for all, is it possible to catch something unpleasant from a public toilet seat?

I quote from a book called *Play Safe: How To Avoid Getting Sexually Transmitted Diseases*, published by the Center For Health Information in Foster City, CA: "Most organisms that transmit sexual diseases need the human body to survive and multiply. Specifically, these organisms require the warmth and moisture found in mucous membranes such as the tissue inside the mouth, vagina and urinary tract. A toilet seat, for the most part, does not provide this type of environment. Crabs and scabies, because they are insects, can survive for long periods of time outside the human body. However, one would have to perch in quite a strange position in order to have one's genitals infected by organisms that might be present on a toilet seat."

chapter eight
The Social Square Dance
(Meeting, Mingling, and Finding Partners)

Ask Isadora

I have been single again for less than two years, but it sure hasn't been the fantasy wonderland I was led to expect. Nearly every man I've been sexual with has some major sexual problem—voyeurism, marathon bangers who both bruise and bore me with hours of bedroom calisthenics, or premature ejaculators. Is it me? Can I do something to avoid this?

Even in fairy tales it's difficult to find something that suits exactly. Look at Goldilocks. Men who poke along, finish too soon, or don't even start may have been perfect partners for somebody else. It could be that you are contributing to this by your selection process. And yes, you can avoid disappointment in the majority of your sexual encounters. Communicate your needs and wants before, during and/or after your connections, and keep in mind that ideal bed partners are created, not (just) made.

Books and articles assure us that the people placing or answering relationship ads are not losers. Are all the ad writers winners? After reading so many ads seeking attractive, slender young women, I wonder if there actually are enough to meet the demand. What happens to all those who are klutzes or fat or disabled or plain or even ugly? What about us losers? Some of us may have lost our youth or our cuteness or our figures or our tans or our hair or our capital or our sight or our grace or our mobility or our self-esteem or our memories or our backhands or our virginity or an election. (I'm an almost 48-year-old fat, feminist woman with a funny nose and no makeup who's too clumsy to dance or cross the street in high heels.) So, what about us losers?

A frequent workshop topic of mine is "Where Can I Find My Valentine?" I usually begin with, "Look at me. If I *believed* all the wants stated by men in the personal ads, I would go right home and put my head under the covers." I, too, am over 40, overweight, and inept in all the California "in" things from skiing to organic gardening. I even (horrors!) smoke. With all this personal disclosure I also want to add that the man is my life is tall, blond, bright and beautiful, everybody's cover-boy concept although I did not choose him for these attributes, and 14 years my junior. He says he's lucky to have me...and I believe him. Anyone who would exclude me from his or her life because my packaging didn't conform to some media-induced image would be shallow indeed, and missing out on the extraordinary experience of my friendship. Do you see what the difference is between you and me? Even at my worst moments, I wouldn't dream of thinking of myself as a loser although someone looking at me might think so. Please consider doing some work on your self-esteem.

I'm an average-looking man of 30 with no special woman in my life. Actually, there are hardly any women in my life at all. I work in a mostly male environment and eat lunch regularly in the company cafeteria. A woman who work there always greets me pleasantly, though our conversations have been limited to the weather and what's on the menu. Yesterday a male co-worker said it's obvious that she's interested in me. The thought never occurred to me. My question is: How can I tell if she, or any woman for that matter, is interested? Maybe I've been missing all kinds of signals.

Some time ago I met a man at a party where I knew no one. We spoke for a few minutes and got separated in the crush. I had no idea whether he was available or interested and no way to find out. I looked for him in the crowd and followed him, "accidentally" bumping into him at least four times. At the end of our last conversation, I enthused effusively about how much I'd enjoyed our meeting, shook his hand warmly, said emphatically how very much I hoped we'd connect again, and gave him my card. He phoned a week later. When our affair was well underway, he confessed how scary it had been for him to initiate the relationship. *Him* initiate? I thought I had done everything short of a nude fandango to demonstrate my eagerness to know him better. This story might serve to indicate that there is no sure way human beings signal potential sexual interest. We are not mating peacocks. She has been friendly and you have been friendly. Someone has got to risk something more to get anything further going. You have no idea how much of a risk she feels she's already made, *if* she has, and neither has your co-worker. You want to play for higher stakes than meatloaf? Nothing ventured, nothing gained.

Last week I attended four social events where the purpose was to meet and mingle with the opposite sex. There were several women I might have liked to talk with, but in no case did they arrive in anything less than packs—groups of two, three, and in one case, seven. It's hard enough for a man to risk being rejected in a social overture, but impossible for me in front of an audience of kibitzers. For instance, if I ask one woman in a group to dance and she refuses, I can't very well ask any other woman in that group since she'd feel like she was second choice. I'm sure I'm not alone in this. Don't women realize how self-defeating it is to travel in groups if they want to meet a man?

Perhaps the prerequisite of running an all-female gauntlet to ask for a lady's favors is the modern-day equivalent of slaying a dragon, jousting in a tournament, or solving The Riddle of the Sphinx. It serves as proof to the object of your attentions that she's worth a risk that would daunt lesser suitors. Actually, I do sympathize with your predicament. Many women will simply not consider going anywhere in public alone, and that's really too bad for all concerned. Having female companions along often inhibits the woman herself, as well as potential suitors. One way to minimize the risk of *en masse* rejection is to survey the lay of the land first. Check out who is moving to the music or talking to folks at the next table for cues as to who is likely to want to dance or willing to speak with a stranger. Making eye contact first, smiling or receiving a smile or some other nonverbal acknowledgement from a woman before approaching her, is usually a good way to increase your chances of receiving a pleasant welcome. Another way is to approach as a person meeting a group of fellow human beings rather than as a fox to the chicken coop. Try "Would any of you care to dance?" or "May I borrow a match from any of you?" Once in conversation with any or all of the women, you can better assess your chances of making one-to-one contact with the preferred member.

What is wrong with these letters (three enclosed) indicative of the seven or eight I've sent in the past year as responses to personal ads? Would Hemingway have been stood up if he were one of 50 or 60 respondents? Of the seven or eight letters I've written like those, not one has elicited a phoned or written response! Is it my handwriting? Does my profession of writer/designer intimidate people? I'm a big boy, so answer candidly: does the enclosed photo rep-

Ask Isadora

resent an entry in the "Best Dogs of San Francisco" contest? I'm at a loss. People make an effort to compose and pay for an ad and then don't even acknowledge receipt of responses. It's their choice, of course, but I'm tapping you for feminine wisdom. Perhaps others have similar complaints.

Your letters seem well-aimed at the ads you enclosed, and your picture shows a man of better-than-average good looks. I don't know what I can add to your letter except "Amen", or in this case, "Ah, women." Women are not the only parties guilty in this regard, however. I'm still smarting from the thundrous silence that greeted a letter I wrote some time back to a man seeking "a very clever, curvaceous woman." I answered with a poem beginning "I am ample of hip." Now that was a good line if I do say so myself. He might have ceded me that. Perhaps he likes tiny tushes and your ladies loathed the favorite movie you mentioned. A postcard to a person who responds to your ad saying thank you for your honesty, your letter, or just for investing the postage stamp money, plus an ambiguous "Perhaps we'll meet some time in the future" if you're not interested, is just common courtesy from anyone to anyone else.

One of the standard lines I seem to be hearing from men lately is "I don't want any involvements or commitments." How can a woman find a meaningful relationship without being threatening to a man?

Anybody whose stated intent is to get something from you that you don't want to give has to be perceived as a threat. You might take such men at their word and look elsewhere for what you want, or back off a bit and lighten up in the hope that there will be an eventual change of heart. There often is. But since you have been forewarned, you can be aware of the risk to your emotions and decide whether this particular man is worth the taking of it.

I am a woman-defined female of 29. The people I usually want to do business with, socialize with, or become intimate with are women. I don't like the term 'lesbian'; it sounds like a geographical designation—"Is she Armenian, Italian or Lesbian?" In fact, I don't like being called by my sexual orientation any more than I would like being defined by my country of origin. My question is: Where can I meet other people, sexual minorities or whatever, where I can just be me without labels?

There are a number of groups listed in the Yellow Pages under Women's Organizations and Services that might interest you. You might want to associate with the gay/bisexual community at large and its supporters. Or you can expand your horizons to see yourself as a member of the human race by volunteering to work for improved literacy, world peace or famine relief. Most organizations with a social cause or philanthropic purpose welcome a willing head, heart and hands without concern for activities occasionally engaged in by other body parts.

After a marriage of twenty years I feel like Alice in Wonderland being single. I've heard about the man shortage for a woman my age, but I see attractive men everywhere. How can I tell if a man I meet is gay?

You can't. Neither can I. If the fact is of importance to you and you're unwilling to let it be revealed in its (or his) own good time, ask. If a man requests or agrees to see you again, that's no guarantee that he's not. If he refuses, it might be comforting to your ego to assume that he is.

Ask Isadora

I'm not a bad-looking guy, but women usually ignore me when I approach them. Could I be too abrupt or ask the wrong questions? What I usually start the conversation with is "Where do you live?" Does that come off as trying too hard?

No, but it is an awkward beginning and obviously doesn't work. My response would be a defensive "Why do you want to know?" Safety is an important consideration for women, and a strange man asking a personal question out of the blue is not conducive to feeling open and friendly. A neutral comment about where you both are ("Nice music" or "This bus is always late"), accompanied by a friendly smile, allows for easier entrance into a give-and-take conversation about music, buses or whatever. It also gives room for a more pleasant brush-off like "Hmmm," which is not necessarily a personal rejection but indicates an unwillingness to have a conversation with a stranger.

I'm a happily married woman of 38 whose only sexual partner has been my husband. Perhaps it's all the magazine articles touting the glories of "sisterhood" over the past years, or maybe it's something in the air of San Francisco since we moved here two years ago. At any rate, while I would not consider endangering my marriage by having an affair with a man, I do dream about an intimate, even sexual, friendship with another woman. I just don't have any idea where to meet such a person, and I'm afraid of scandalizing any of the women I do know by what they might feel is an improper advance. Any suggestions?

I'm seeing more personal ads these days reflecting situations like yours. Sometimes it's in the context of the married couple seeking a female third. Sometimes it's just as you describe, an additional secret liaison. So, perhaps the personal ads are one way to begin. You might look for women-oriented meetings or events such as a women's craft fair or concert, for example, or discussion groups on women's issues. As for exploring the sexual possibilities with an existing friend, sometimes it helps to create a conducive context. An evening of hot-tubbing, a trip to an erotic movie, or an overnight camp-out with an offer to exchange massages, can provide the time and privacy and foster the kind of intimate conversational revelations that may lead where you might like to go without undue risk on your part.

At a concert the other evening, the young woman in the row in front of me turned around several times to smile at me. Should I have spoken to her?

"Should" is a very unproductive word. You certainly *could* have.

It might have been that your fly was open. It also might have been that she found you attractive and that was as blatant a come-on as she could muster. And now you'll never know. Make a resolution to act on a positive assumption next time it happens.

Regarding the shortage of men for older women: Women's incomes average 60% of men's. If it weren't for financial considerations, younger women would probably concentrate much more on men of roughly their own age. All other things being equal, everyone would prefer a lover with a relatively beautiful body. Surveys show that for men this is a much more important consideration than it is for women. For women, financial considerations are usually more important. It logically

Ask Isadora

follows that as far as lasting relationships go, older men with money are going to get more of the younger women than older women will get younger men. When older women do get younger men, it is usually a temporary relationship based largely on lust, expediency, or money. If women's incomes are ever raised to those of men, it may spell the death of marriage. Statistics show that the more money a woman makes, the less likely she is to be married, whereas the less money a man makes, the less likely he is to be married. Also, the more money a man makes, the more likely he is to be married and the more likely he is to have extramarital affairs!

If we grant the above inequities as so, what are you doing about it? My younger lusty, impecunious, and opportunistic companion and I (an aging, sagging, graying, experienced older woman), are doing our best...but we can't change the world single-handedly. We need some co-operation from you letter writers out there. No more complaints now. Let's hear it for some action! How about declaring this "Men, Take a Same Age or Older Woman To Lunch (Or Bed)" Week!

I am hoping you might be able to steer me in the right direction. I am single, and finishing school while looking for work. I am somewhat middle-of-the-road: I like to have friends, but am not what you'd call a groupie. I am somewhat conservative and dependable, but still like to fool around. I like to go out drinking and dancing, but the people you meet might not necessarily be the greatest. The couple of church groups I have tried were full of people chasing some mystique or who were there to use up a Sunday night. Any suggestions as to where I might find a "support group"?

Isadora Alman

Support groups usually form around a particular problem area such as smoking, self-defeating relationships, or excessive spending. It seems to me what you're looking for is a compatible friend or two. There are such things as men's groups whose purpose is supporting men's relations with other men. There are similar groups for both men and women whose focus is on the dilemmas of making connections. These groups are usually advertised in growth-oriented magazines and newspapers. Look under such headings as Relationships, Social Clubs, Personal Growth, Sexuality, or some special interest of yours like dancing or computers.

There are quality, legitimate social clubs for straight males and females, gay men, bi men, lesbian women, Jewish singles, Christian singles, herpes sufferers, younger men/older women, over 50s, and just about every other type of single person you can imagine. They are offered numerous attractive services from travel packages to wine tastings where they can meet and mingle. We are a young upscale couple who reject denial of desires outside our relationship and deal with them by sharing these desires with liberal, sincere friends. But once you're a couple society offers the choice of suppressing your interests, or labeling you as a sleazy "swinger," left to using grotesque street tabloids to find persons with which to satisfy your disgusting urges! We'd like you to publish the names, if they exist, of any legitimate social clubs or placement services that help liberal, open-minded and normal couples to meet like-minded persons interested in sincere and possibly intimate relationships.

If you were looking for congenial couples with whom to share a winter ski cabin you would ask among your friends likely to be interested in the sport, or go to organizations of skiers hoping to winnow out those members you particularly like. Sharing sex is just a degree or two more intimate than sharing living quarters, and you may have to conduct your search in precisely the same manner—discreetly among the people you know, and at commercial gatherings of swingers. Sleazy, like normal, is a highly subjective term. PEP, Polyfidelitous Educational Productions, publishes information and networking opportunities. Write them at P.O. Box 6306, Captain Cook, Hawaii 96704-6306. They may be able to steer you toward clubs or groups closer to home.

The most ideal living and loving arrangement I can imagine is several people in what I guess most people would call a "group marriage" or an "extended family." I live alone in a pretty isolated area and I have trouble meeting people. How could I begin to realize my dream?

As in working toward any goal—one step at a time. Most of us have trouble finding even one acceptable partner and accustoming him or her to our ways of living and loving...or negotiating a mutually suitable accommodation. You might begin by looking for personal ads placed by existing "families," couples or groups, placing an ad yourself, or concentrating your search within such organizations as PEP which support and encourage explorations into unconventional living arrangements.

I am an attractive young man. I would like to be able to approach women in public places, but I'd just as soon not approach women who aren't interested. I know eye contact is a very important part of body language, but I haven't mastered the basic vocabulary. If a woman is looking in my direction she could be just looking around, checking me out, flirting inconsequentially, inviting me over, or directing her attention to someone behind me. Are there ways to reduce the ambiguity of such a situation? How can I develop some skills without initiating misunderstandings rather than friendships?

Initial social encounters are always ambiguous, that's part of their charm—playing with that "will she?" or "might he?" possibility. Even a broad wink aimed in your direction could indicate a speck in a woman's eye rather than a lascivious come-on. Many women just cannot be approached comfortably in a public place for a variety of reasons, none of which would have a thing to do with your skills in body language. She might be with someone, have an old-fashioned sense of propriety, or simply be afraid to accept gestures of any kind from strangers. If you are willing to risk a brush-off nonetheless, maneuvering yourself to within commenting distance of the woman in question and then making some innocuous social pleasantry about the common situation you find yourself in—"Marvelous concert, don't you think?"—is the gentlest way of exploring her interest in engaging in conversation with you. In the matter of learning about body language, experience is the very best teacher and willingness to take risks the very best method of scholarship.

I am a man in my late 50s, divorced, semi-retired. I have no desire to remain single. I am looking, as I say in the personal ads I've placed, for a woman who is "warm, has an outgoing personality, is financially independent, healthy, physically active, and fairly well educated." Am I asking too much? Most of the women who reply to my ads are divorced single mothers in low-paying uncertain jobs, just barely surviving. I know that unfortunately many women fall into the low end of the financial spectrum, and I am not proud of being a member of a society where this is so. But since I am paying alimony and continue to support several children in college, I do not want to divide what I have left again or to give up the few advantages I can enjoy after 33 years in public service—travel, enjoying the arts, living simply but without financial worry. Unless I pay all the costs (travel, meals, entertainment), the women I meet can rarely go out with me. While dating I don't mind this, but in the long run I don't want to be financially responsible for anyone else. Am I unreasonable or am I doing something wrong?

Your requirements in a prospective wife sound neither unreasonable nor unmeetable, but a change of tactics is definitely in order. You can continue to singlehandedly, and grudgingly, right the economic inequities inflicted by other men on the women you date, or do one or several of the following: Using your tried and true methods you can date poor women *only* if they are ambitious—those back in school, for instance, or in entry-level jobs that they intend using as a stepping stone. You can wine and dine them or more often gear your times together to exchanging home cooking or attending free events. You can rewrite your ads to emphasize a financially equal marriage in the future, so that more likely women respond. You can advertise in media more likely to be read by the women you seek than the alternative newspapers you mention. And, you can use the activities you enjoy such as travel and entertainment events to meet the women who have the means to do the same—the ones that are there alone or with a friend. Broaden your outlook a bit and dare to dream. There are thousands of women out there who want exactly what you do.

My marriage of fifteen years ended a year ago when my husband left me for another woman, his secretary. I'm still very angry. I would like to get on with my life, perhaps begin dating again, but I don't know where to begin. Any suggestions?

My first suggestion would be a support, therapy, or discussion group of people in your situation and/or a good counselor (who often run such groups) specializing in letting go of anger, recovering from a separation, and learning social skills. The dating and mating rituals have changed a great deal in some respects over the past fifteen years, and in many other respects not at all. If you will be seeking the company of men approximately your age, they will often be in the same situation as you are—hurting from a past break-up and trying to resuscitate rusty social graces. A support group of newly single preferably one with both women and men, offers a safe, comfortable setting in which to meet some new friends and to learn and try out new ways of thinking and behaving.

I'm a bisexual white male, 90% straight, 10% gay. I'm a friendly, intelligent college grad, and not bad looking. However, I am dull, low-energy, and socially and sexually withdrawn. Emotionally I'm dead inside, and I'm afraid the truth is I'm very boring. I'm mostly a loner and have to be by myself a lot. I've been this way despite years of psychotherapy. I've come to accept that I'll be this way for a long time, possibly forever. Despite the way I am, I have made a few good friends over the years, so I know it is possible for me to have relationships with people. I wonder if you have any suggestions where I might meet a woman, or perhaps a man, who is on my energy level.

James Bugantal, a Humanist psychotherapist, defines the purpose of therapy as increasing the experience of being alive, particularly inward aliveness. He equates successful therapy with obtaining "an enlarged sense of one's being and power in life." Not having met you, I am in no position to argue with your self-assessment of dull and boring. I do know, however, that all of us structure our world and the experiences we have in life by our belief system. If you believe, for instance, that all redheaded women are gold-diggers, you will find "proof" in every one you meet, redefining a gold-digging brunette as having reddish hair in order to substantiate your position. So, first of all, stick with therapy; or find a different, more effective, therapist who can help you get in touch with and enlarge upon your sense of aliveness (that which attracted and bound to you those friends you do have.) Second, explore various discussion, encounter, therapy groups. The more people you meet, the more you will have to chose potential partners from. Concentrating only on people who match your own low energy and esteem could only yield a dreary relationship indeed. Someone whose energy compliments rather than duplicates your style might be a better match. Super-high energy people often long for a mate who is stable and unemotional. That way each can assist the other in effecting a happier balance.

I am a straight, attractive, reasonably well-adjusted young woman who has not been involved in an intimate relationship with a man in over three years. I am actively "trying to put myself out there," but I keep coming up empty and increasingly lonely and depressed. What suggestions do you have for women like me, neither barfly nor jockette types, who are sincerely interested in meeting quality men? I am not so cynical (yet) to believe that they really don't exist. I'm wary of singles groups but at this point I'm willing to try just about anything. Are there any particular organizations, clubs, which in your opinion are worthwhile?

If your particular definition of "quality man" is an East Coast-bred Ivy League creative type, for example, then any group, club, party, etc. which featured a huge selection of these would be worthwhile, while any that didn't wouldn't. So part of the process for you is choosing where and how to spend your search time. Start with people you know—friends, co-workers, relatives, and put out to them a sense of what you want. People generally love to matchmake. Ask for suggestions from acquaintances who successfully found a mate. See what classes are available near you in tax management, wine tasting, folk dancing—something of interest to you and likely to be of interest to those you seek. Don't neglect newspapers as a source of ideas, particularly the alternative press and free publications. Check out the personal ads, the social services and clubs and the calendar section for events you might like, and try whatever looks promising at least once; even go alone! Find ways to enjoy the process of mate hunting by playing smarter rather than working harder.

I am a straight white male looking for very sexually active girls who desire a lot of various cultures' sex, like Greek. I've tried swinger magazines, but there's a lot of bullshit in them like girls responding with "send money for pictures." The dating and bar scene doesn't do it for me. I'm hoping that you will

Ask Isadora

direct me to a club of sincere girls who will be what I'm looking for.

Honey, you are whistling from the same aperture where you desire your culture. There is no such thing as a hangout for sexually ravenous women ready to welcome any and all takers out of the goodness of their hearts. Most women would prefer to think that any lust directed their way is inspired by their beauty, charm or personality rather than their being endowed by nature with an orifice suited to your needs of the moment. You will, however, increase your chances of getting laid without the necessity of lengthy or extravagant courtship rituals by looking for partners where the nature of the event is specifically geared to sexual connection—commercial swinging houses, for instance.

You are right, Isadora, when you say there are many single healthy women out there looking for a solid honest relationship. I am incarcerated, but once I let it be known I was willing to write to interested females some of the mail responses and photographs I received make even me blush. Three women I have never met—one from Nevada, one from Oregon, and one from San Diego—are coming to meet me Friday, Saturday and Sunday of next week, and there are more who hope to. All this with only four or five letters and an hour or so of phone conversation. Hey, I'm not complaining. I just wonder what the problem is when I keep reading about guys on the outside with a lot more going for them who can't connect with a woman.

Either you write the world's most knock-yer-socks-off personal ad, or all these single, honest, solid women who are responding to you are not all that healthy. Some women love playing Martyr and others love the role of Messiah. For some, the appeal is the "macho" glamour of a convict lover (some women chase truckers or cops for the same reason). To others there is a special thrill in the amount of ardor and attention a lover who has little else to do but fantasize about them will direct their way. In the same way teenagers often fall in love with movie stars, some may see having a lover in lockup as the perfect solution for what they crave—all that hot fantasy of love and longing without the dirty, icky reality of an in-the-flesh sexual relationship. I have no doubt that you have something of value to offer these women, but let's face it, it is limited. You don't say when or if you are scheduled for release, but if it's not in the near future a romance with a jail inmate is likely to prove even more frustrating for a woman than the time-honored one with a married man. There are women who thrive on doing that number, too.

Reader response: *Your comments on the women who engage in prisoner correspondence looked right on target to me. I recently received an account of one woman's experience in writing to, and later marrying, a prisoner which concludes: "I learned that a person can say anything he wants on a piece of paper, but his actions are what count; you will never never know what these actions are until he is on the street." The subject comes up often in our magazine, not only about prisoners but other correspondents as well.*

This letter writer is the editor and publisher of a magazine for people who write letters on a wide range of interests and who enjoy meeting each other (often solely) through the mail. (SASE to The Letter Exchange, P.O. Box 6218, Albany, CA 94706.) The Summer 1988 copy of their newsletter

Ask Isadora

bears this editorial caveat: "Caution. Talking to strangers invariably involves risk. Since this magazine is sold without restrictions, available to anyone, we have no way to judge the integrity or intentions of its buyers....Please go slowly, particularly at the start. Get to know your correspondents. Easy does it." Sounds like a sign that could well be posted at every public or private gathering.

I have a problem—perhaps. I am a healthy gay male of 40 who has perversely gained a desire to have sex with a woman. I am interested in a sexual experience, not a relationship. A commercial transaction might well be what's appropriate, but I don't want an off-the-street liaison. Maybe there's a lesbian somewhere with a complementary state of mind. How does one like me find such a partner?

You are not alone in your quandary. There are a great many hetero men who are also looking for a sexual experience without a concomitant relationship. You might look into meeting an open-minded partner in organizations with a non-traditional outlook. You might consider being with a sexual surrogate (through referral from a savvy therapist), or you might consider placing a personal ad. There are a number of women—lesbian, bisexual or straight, who might enjoy playing Henry Higgins to your Eliza Doolittle.

I am a very attractive single female in my early 30s. Frequently I am the recipient of whistles and waves on the street or in my car. However, in the past two years I have had a dramatic decrease in dates. I am a very active individual. I don't stay home a lot and am involved in commu-

nity affairs. People call me a very nice person, but I never get asked out. I have tried asking men out and they have been successful one-time dates. They don't call me back. I am wondering if men in general are afraid of sustaining a long-term relationship with someone who has good moral values, is intelligent and reasonably successful.

I don't think one can damn men as an aggregate, although this might be true of the men you have been meeting recently. First, though, I would be inclined to look closely at, one, your expectations about dating and courtship ("they're supposed to ask me out; they're supposed to follow up"), and, two, your demeanor. Perhaps there is something about you that is offputting to prospective boyfriends—you might seem aloof or overly eager. Helpful information of that nature could come from some trusted friends of either sex, a good interactional counselor, or, best yet, a support/discussion group on men's and women's issues.

A recent article you mentioned on your radio show dealt with learning how to form friendships, not necessarily sexual ones. Would you be willing to say more about that?

I was quoting something reprinted from the *New York Times*: "Research into how children perceive popularity has shown that until they reach adolescence, few children understand the role their own behavior plays in how many friends they have. Children will tell you that people who have a lot of friends are just lucky." My comment was, what makes the good researcher think that this belief is limited to children? The number of intimate connections in a person's life is related to how good a

Ask Isadora

friend that person *is*. If you're nice to be around, people are going to want to be around you. The skills of being a good listener, acknowledging others for their accomplishments, refraining from excessive complaining and the like are learnable skills, easier for some than for others, I grant, but not impossible to acquire for most humans over the age of four.

I'm considered attractive, a person with a career position, and an incurable romantic with so much love to give. I'm a 24-year-old guy with a pretty basic problem: I can't seem to find Ms. Right. I've tried virtually everything. The bar scene just doesn't work for me. Trying to meet women at Safeway doesn't either. They're either married, engaged, or just there for the cantaloupes. I have tried the ads, and I have made true and meaningful friendships, but nothing more. Does Ms. Right really exist, Isadora, or is she a product of my imagination?

It depends on what you imagine, and on how detailed your Wish List is. While happy couples have been known to begin at bars, supermarkets and through personal ads (which have a better success rate than the former sources), statistics indicate that most couples meet through continuing contact—such as classmates, work colleagues, fellow club members, etc. The reason is that in this way people can gradually see beyond a well-rounded *this* or a muscle-toned *that* to other, more lasting qualities like a happy disposition, fine intelligence, or mutually compatible interests and goals. While I'm certainly not one to pooh-pooh the power of sexual attraction, Ms. Right, when found, usually has more to recommend her than a fortuitous arrangement of idealized body parts. I know many people, me among them, who are happily involved with, and hence, attracted to as well, an individual who is "not their physical type at all." These pairings would never have resulted from a shouted come-on in a noisy bar or a once-over at the cantaloupe counter.

chapter nine
Communication Is the Best Lubrication
(Communication Techniques)

Ask Isadora

I've heard you lecture on several occasions, and I know how much you encourage clear communication as a part of good sex. I'm afraid of hurting my partner's feelings, though, if I ask him to do something other than the usual. Please give me some specific suggestions on positive ways I can encourage him to do what pleases me.

One method is non-verbal communication, which is what sex is anyway. Arrange to have whatever body parts need to be there in the position you want them to be, placing a hand or mouth or whatever where you want it and guiding it in your preferred rhythm. Murmur approving noises when it's being done right. If it's more complicated than that, you might suggest doing something untried in a spirit of adventure. Look up over dinner and say mischievously, "I've been having this fantasy about..." If they never let you back into that restaurant, well, good restaurants are easier to find than loving playmates.

I am a 28 year-old-single woman with basically one problem for you. I have a difficult time achieving an orgasm. Now, the problem is not with me—it's with my partners. I enjoy all aspects of lovemaking, but my partners become frustrated and feel inadequate when they feel they have not satisfied me. We talk about the situation and I explain it will come in time (no pun intended!), but this situation seems to hurt their fragile male egos. My last relationship ended suddenly with the explanation that we just "didn't cut it" in bed and his ego just couldn't deal with that anymore. I am now involved with someone else, and he seems disturbed about me not achieving orgasm. I don't want this to be a problem, but what can I do? I am almost to the point of faking, but I'm sure that would just bring on another problem.

The easiest solution to your by-no-means-easily-resolved concern is for you to learn to have fairly reliable orgasms on your own by some method, and then to teach that method to your partner. There is always the possibility that he won't be able to cope with your preferred method—be it hand, mouth, vibrator or convoluted coital position—and will be disgruntled still, but at least you'd have the satisfaction of an occasional orgasm. Talk about the fact that your responses are something you've been comfortable with and hope in time that he will too. Do give your partner lots of positive reinforcement ("I love it when you..." "It really excites me when we..."), so that he will feel appreciated as a lover even without the standard accolade of your orgasm.

I guess I'm an affable sort. I can talk to strangers easily. I have no trouble putting together a volleyball game on the beach or doing business development for the branch bank where I work. It's only when I meet someone I'm really attracted to that I seem to fall apart and forget every piece of small talk I've ever heard or used. What can I do to use whatever natural charm I might have at the times it counts most?

If it isn't one of Murphy's Laws, it's surely one of Alman's that the quality of a performance is usually in inverse proportion to how much quality matters. Are you more likely to shoot a hole-in-one while entertaining a prospective client who's a golf nut or when you're fooling around by yourself on a makeshift green? Yep, right. One way to reduce your anxiety when meeting Person Wonderful is to keep on mutteringly reminding yourself that you've been successful in meeting people a thousand times before, and underneath the stunning exterior is a human being just like all the others you've managed to charm. It's the old "puts his pants (or her pantyhose) on one leg at a time" ploy. Another method is to own up to what's going on with you and hope that it will be taken as the compliment it is: "I'm usually pretty glib, but your good looks seem to stop my tongue in its tracks." In the happy event that person finds you equally attractive, saying anything that comes to mind about the here and now, even "My, the walls are perpendicular tonight," will be gratefully seized upon as a conversational opener, since the other person is no doubt wrestling with the same dilemma.

My lady friend keeps calling me by her last lover's name. Our names aren't at all similar and, from what I hear, neither are we. She does have the grace to apologize when it happens, but after six months it's beginning to bug me. What do you think it means, and how can I get her to quit?

It could mean that she'd prefer to be with Lover #1. (That's what you were afraid you might hear, right?) It could also mean that she's a creature of habit, and that for a long enough time for it to become a reflex action, Man At Her Side was addressed as _____, which she continues to use in the same manner as some doting aunts continue to address a balding 55-year-old-executive as "Bubba." You could tell her how disturbed you feel when she continues to slip up. You could invent a private nickname she wouldn't dare call anyone else, like Lover Lips or Hammer Hips. You might make a joke of it when it happens by calling her some name other than hers, perhaps your mother's. Your friend could consider the somewhat affected but undeniably useful ploy of referring to all within her circle of familiars by some unisex endearment. That works very well for me, except on occasions when a comment directed to "Sweetie" elicits responses from my daughter, my lover, my best friend and my cat!

My wife and I have been invited to spend a weekend at the country home of a couple we met at a jazz club we all belong to. We were told there would be "other congenial couples" present. Something in the way the invitation was extended leads me to infer that these people may be "swingers." I can't very well ask if group sex is part of the weekend's planned entertainment, but if it is, I'd like to be prepared. Is there some sort of protocol for these things?

Like the rules for charades, different customs prevail among different groups of players. I'd certainly suggest sharing your suspicions with your wife and seeing how she feels about it. You two can then make whatever agreements are necessary to your comfort. These can range from "Let's leave at the first drop of a bathing suit" to "Enjoy yourself and I'll meet you by the car Sunday afternoon." You can then present a united front to your hosts and wing it from there. Most swingers are easygoing, and if any rules prevail across group lines, they are that "No, thank you" means just that with no further explanations required, and that any sort of coercion beyond "Try it (me, us), you might like it" is considered extremely bad form.

I am a 25-year-old bisexual woman. I left my hometown seven years ago and have not been back since. I recently received a phone call from someone I went to high school with, asking me if she could come here for a visit because she needed to talk to me about something important. I can't stop her from making the trip, and I must admit I'm curious. The

Ask Isadora

only reason I can see for her to come out is to come out, if you know what I mean. My question is: Why me? I've always been a private person and not discussed my personal business with anyone; not then, not now.

Neither of us can guess the purpose of this woman's visit. Once you hear her out, then you'll know. Listening to whatever she wants to tell you does not imply a contract of exchanging intimacies. You can certainly ask her why she chose you as a confidante. Maybe she wants to know how you managed to move away from home and avoid returning for seven years. It is quite a feat.

I'm 35 and I have been living with this man for a few months now. When I'm in the mood for sex I think I communicate that to him very clearly. He either doesn't hear me or doesn't understand me, and I don't want to have to come right out and say "Do you want to?" How can I get him to respond?

There's an exercise I do in some of my workshops. A couple sits back to back and one of them says, "Please listen to me." The other responds in one of three ways: "I can't hear you," "I don't understand you," or "No." This dialogue is repeated over and over for several minutes. Most people say that the feeling of intense frustration they experience when doing this exercise is uncomfortably familiar. You might ask your lover at some neutral time how, in the future, he would like you to let him know when you are interested. A small quirky smile is a neon sign for some people. Others prefer a more direct method of seduction, like "Let's!" One possibility is that he both hears and understands you and is saying "No" with the same subtle communication methods you use. You're not risking an outright invitation, so he's not risking an outright refusal.

Isadora Alman

My lover is an alcoholic. We've been seeing each other for almost three years. Frankly, being involved with him has become more trouble than he's worth. Is there any way to end the relationship without hurting him? I don't want to add to his problems.

Being rejected always hurts—drunk, sober, or in the fuzzy state in between. If you are firm in your resolve that this is what you want to do—and you will need to be firm for both of your sakes—choose a time that he's likely to hear you and tell him how you feel. If his drinking is an important factor in your disenchantment, he needs to hear that too. Write it down in a letter and mail it to him if you can't face a personal confrontation, but be sure to include the positive things about him that kept you hanging around all this time. I presume he's aware of support groups like AA if he wants to make any changes, but you may want to know there are affiliate groups for people involved with problem drinkers that can offer you some emotional backup in your decision. It is not your fault he drinks and will not be your fault if he continues to do so.

I'm very much in love with a woman I've been seeing for several months and I tell her often. When I say "I love you," her usual response is "I'm glad," or "Thank you," but she never says she loves me.

Are you asking me whether she does or not? May I respectfully suggest you redirect this to the only person who could possibly give you a satisfactory response. Remember Isadora's Dictum: Never ask a direct question to which you are not prepared to hear an honest answer. Consider telling her instead that you would like to know how she feels about you, a reasonable request under the circumstances.

Ask Isadora

I'm a single mother of two boys, 12 and 16. The younger one asks me more personal questions than my gynecologist and already knows more about life than I did when I was married. The older boy blushes if anyone so much as mentions sex in his presence, and turns away all my best efforts to open any discussion on the topic. I would like to make sure that each of my sons knows whatever is necessary to be healthy and well-informed, but I'm afraid I'm telling too much to the little one and not enough to his brother. Help.

What might look like prurient interest on the 12-year-old's part could be intellectual curiosity, and therefore devoid of the paralyzing embarrassment it has for your teenager, for whom sex has emotional reality. This situation may also be the result of individual differences in communication style, which you all should recognize in yourselves and each other. If your younger son gets too personal in his search for information, assure him that you will be as respectful of the privacy of his sexual feelings as you insist he be of yours. Set your limits: "Many men do this, many women feel that, but what I do and feel is my personal affair." I'm sure you've had occasion in your 16 years together to tell your older son things he doesn't want to listen to, even if it was about getting a haircut or turning down his stereo. Acknowledge his reticence and, giving him the same excellent reason you gave me, forge ahead anyway. Recently, with his parents' permission, I gave copies of *The Joy of Sex* and my own book, *Aural Sex & Verbal Intercourse,* to the son of friends as a bar mitzvah present. His rather ungracious response was, "Aw, I already know all this stuff." His mother tells me, however, that a larger than usual number of his pals stopped by the following week to "look over his presents and stuff." How interesting can bonds and pen and pencil sets be? Offering books or other resources, such as the phone number of a sex information hot line, lets him know he has options other than talking things over with (shudder) Mom.

I know this might sound like a line as old as farmers' daughter jokes, but I'm writing about someone else's problem, not mine. I have a friend with a hang-up about sex. I don't think she has much sexual experience, if any. She's in her late 20s and she looks uncomfortable if anyone mentions sex or makes sexual allusions. Even though I'm a heterosexual man, I don't have any designs on her personally. I just care enough about her to worry that she's missing out on a great deal of pleasure in life. Is there anything I can do or say to enlighten her? Would this be better coming from another woman?

Changing someone else's attitude or behavior for them is generally a losing proposition, but the world abounds with teachers and preachers who feel otherwise, so it may not be entirely hopeless. Saying to her directly what you have written to me may be the opening for a productive discussion. If she opens up enough to you to admit ignorance of the subject, fears, lack of self-esteem, or a dearth of suitable potential partners, you can help by recommending books, support or discussion groups, counselling, or an introduction to some of your other friends, male or female, as her wishes dictate. At the very least she will know that someone cares about her happiness, a very comforting thought to anyone.

My partner of two years seems to be increasingly unhappy in our relationship. When I asked him about it all he said was that I wasn't paying him enough attention. What do you think that means?

Ask Isadora

I know what it means when I say it, and I make sure the person to whom I direct such a complaint knows too, as well as exactly how they might go about rectifying it: "I feel ignored when you read the newspaper at the table," or "We haven't made love for what feels like a terribly long time," or "I'd really like to be surprised with flowers every once in a while." See if your partner will say something more helpful about the times, occasions, and ways he would like your attention. Trying to make another person happy when they don't define some ways and means of doing so is like trying to bake a chocolate cake "just like Mom's" with no recipe.

I am 26 and single. I do volunteer work several hours a week in my parish church. My co-worker is a plump lady in her 40s. She is not bad looking at all. I'd go for her anytime. Last week she wore a skirt with the hemline above her knees and an open slit on one side. When she sat down on a sofa to talk to me I got a clear view all the way up her thighs. I was wondering whether to put my hands on her. Do you think she was looking for love or sexual intercourse?

While it is quite clear what you were looking *at*, I have no idea what she might have been looking for. If you think she is issuing a sexual invitation to you by wearing clothing you find provocative or by sitting immodestly, there are better ways of checking that out than by grabbing. I suggest inviting her for a drink after work. If, after some private conversation outside of church, you still aren't sure what she wants, tell her you find her attractive or her clothing arousing. Her reaction to your words should indicate whether or not her behavior was intentional.

My wife seems to enjoy sex. She participates enthusiastically whenever I initiate it, but she never starts things herself. How can I get her to be more forthcoming?

I don't think one can successfully "get" another to be or do other than what she is or does. What you can do is tell her how you feel and what you want her to do about it. Then she can hear you and respond, either by doing as you wish or stating her reasons for not doing so. At the very least, you will then have an honest intimate discussion with your wife going rather than a covert game of wishing and manipulation.

"Let's have lunch sometime." I know it has become somewhat of a social cliché, but what does it really mean? Is it, in fact, an invitation, or a polite social noise like "How are you?"

Like "Sure I love you, baby," it can mean a variety of things depending on the speaker and the situation. If it's tossed in your direction by someone with whom you would like to get together again, simply suggest a date. You might also say, "I'd love to. I'll call you." Then, unless you want to perpetuate the practice of insincere social noises, call.

I have been invited to a big family celebration to take place over the holidays in my mid-Western hometown. Of course, I'll be bringing my wife of 14 months. I know my mother will insist on our staying with her, no doubt in the very bedroom in which I grew up. My problem is that I simply cannot imagine making love with my wife under the listening ears of my mother. The thought of it actually makes me go limp. We plan to stay a week and I'm sure my wife will comment if we don't make love during that time. What can I tell her?

The truth—lightly, lovingly, and without any heavy Freudian overtones. If it's a really big deal to her, rather than an amusing quirk of yours she's willing to humor, you might consider staying at a motel. If risking your mother's hurt feelings on that score is also terrible to contemplate, maybe you and your wife might make a game of trying to find time and a place to get it on together somewhere in town, a borrowed car, while your mother is out shopping, or in a shared shower. Where there's a will, there's a way.

I am a woman who likes to have my toes sucked and licked. I learned this from a lover who is no longer in my life. There have been several since him, but unfortunately no one else has initiated this delightful game. I don't know how to ask for it because of the potential implication of subjugation (kissing a person's feet). That really isn't the point for me. I just like the sensation of tongue on my toes. How can I introduce this to a new man without his making more of it than I mean?

You could do it to him, and, regardless of his response, use that situation to let him know of your desires. ("Oh, don't you like it? I just love that sensation when it's done to me.") Another subtle way to introduce some idiosyncratic sexplay into a relationship is to arrange a bet wherein the prize is 15 minutes of pleasure in the manner of one's choice. ("Wanna bet George will tell that joke about the penguins at the party tonight? If he doesn't, you win 15 minutes of uninterrupted delight. Your choice. I'm sure he'll tell it, though, and if I'm right, wait till you see what I want.")

Lately I'm meeting women who are cold fish, interested in stimulation to orgasm, but uninterested in setting the mood or in heightening sexual communication. You know, the things that slowly and subtly build up layers of arousal to the level where just a few fingers brushing over a part of the body can be almost orgasmic. Can you suggest any ways to get a woman more interested in sensuality?

Some people, men or women, want meat and potatoes with salt, pepper, and ketchup. Others will rhapsodize about three teensy globules of fish eggs on a toast triangle as a culinary masterpiece. Sexual subtlety is an acquired taste, as is caviar, and some people find it not worth acquiring. More often than not, it seems to be males who are accused of wanting to get it up, in, off, and over. True or not, any new partner needs to become acquainted with your preferred sexual pace. It may be that the women you're meeting have been conditioned by previous partners to efficiency over delicacy, and need time to readjust. If not, quickies can be fun, so consider trading off.

My new lover is a sweet guy who seems eager to please me in every way. Unfortunately, when it comes to sex he's just not doing things right—for me, anyway. How can I tell him?

Nicely and clearly: "What really turns me on is when you do this just like this. Give me your hand (or whatever part is involved here) and let me show you." It's frustrating for both of you if you lie there hoping he'll eventually stumble across the secret. You can draw a follow-the-dot game onto your skin or conduct a treasure hunt with written clues secreted about your body. You might even invent a bedtime game of charades ("Sounds like...") But there just is no way of letting someone know something without telling them. If your lover is as eager to please as you say, he will probably be delighted to have such information as long as it's imparted

Ask Isadora

in the tender tones of lover to lover rather than those of a drill sergeant to a raw recruit.

On every gift-giving occasion since we were married almost two years ago, my husband has surprised me with an intimate sex-oriented present—a night garment smaller than my bathing suit, some creams and lotions labeled "love balms," and now some silly book on how to keep the sizzle in your marriage. He's obviously trying to tell me something, but whenever I introduce the subject of our sex life in a straightforward manner, he becomes uncomfortable and changes the subject. What more can I do to open communications?

You have already done the obvious by introducing the subject of your sex life in a straightforward manner. Perhaps what's needed is to change the manner of your manner, to warmly encourage rather than confront. "I want to talk to you about our sex life" usually summons the same set of feelings that "The principal would like to see you in his office" did in your youth: Uh oh. Try bringing out one of your gifts and asking in a mildly puzzled and encouraging tone, "I'm sure you had something in mind when you gave me this. Could we discuss whatever you thought this might bring about? I know that it's difficult for you, but if there is something you want that you're not getting from me, I'm afraid you are going to have to be more explicit. I would like to make you happy." Keep trying. It's usually worth it.

My daughter, who is 12, told me that a man on the train exposed himself to her and a girlfriend when they were seated across from him. I was horrified, but she seemed to find the episode funny. How should I handle this?

Since she was apparently not in danger, your daughter's reaction seems quite healthy. Most people who expose themselves in public do so because they expect or hope for a particular reaction—desire, horror, upset, but hardly ever laughter. I can't think of a more "withering" response. Of course you need to remind her of ways to insure her safety, like not traveling alone in unpopulated areas or talking to strangers in cars. Encourage her to walk away at the least sign of suspicious behavior and to report disturbing activities to the nearest police or adult in charge. Since she was not upset in this case, I wouldn't encourage her to become so by making too much of the incident.

My bedroom wall is also the bathroom wall of the apartment next door which a young couple recently rented. Apparently they take baths together, because I am able to hear long intimate conversations, probably amplified by the bathroom tiles. Is there any way I can let them know this without embarrassment?

Miss Manners' dictum, that a lady or gentleman is deaf to noises which occur when others are using the bathroom, is a good one. It sounds like the embarrassment you want to avoid is yours. I suggest suffering it in silence. It's probably a great deal less than that which would be suffered by someone finding out that while supposedly enjoying the privacy of their own bathroom...they are not.

My work at a museum reception desk brings me into contact with people from all over the world, especially in the summer tourist season. I notice enormous variations in conversational "styles." Some people avert their eyes when I'm talking to them, others stare into mine. Some people need to crowd very close, some touch, some smile. I enjoy noticing all these different ways of social intercourse, but I feel I'd learn a lot more if there was some recognizable pattern. Are these individual differences I'm seeing or are they cultural ones?

Both. People vary within cultural norms. For example, look at the American custom of the introductory handshake. Teachers of social skills suggest a firm, brief clasping of hands with the elder, female, and or more prestigious person making the initial outreach. By no means do all Americans know to do this, or bother, or do it "correctly" if and when they do. Yet in most business and social settings many of us judge others and are judged ourselves by how well we adhere to this "norm."

Is there a polite way of letting someone dear to you know that his or her standards of personal hygiene are not as you would like them to be?

If there are, "Yo, stinky!" is not one of them. One method might be offering a suggested explanation at the same time you pose the problem: "You smell different than you usually do. Are you using some new shampoo or skin cream?" When questioned, you might then reluctantly admit that no, you really can't say that you do like it, whatever it is, and you prefer whatever he/she used before. Another approach is to praise the obvious: "I am really turned on by the scent of your body when you step right out of the shower," or "Let's take a bath before we go to bed. I love the feel of our not-quite-dry bodies bumping together under the covers." Being told what pleases, one can infer what does not. When all else fails, be loving, gentle, apologetic for any hurt feelings, and direct nevertheless.

Isadora Alman

I am 37 years old and I attend a clinic once a year to have a pap smear. Last time I was there the person examining me said in an offhand way, "Did you know your vaginal wall is collapsing?" She didn't explain further and I guess I was too stunned to ask. Now I don't know whether I should have it checked out by a private doctor or not. What exactly does that mean?

The only one who could say *exactly* is a medically knowledgeable person familiar with the walls of your vagina. When faced with a diagnosis, whether of one's person or one's car, I always ask three very pertinent questions: "What do you recommend I do about what you have told me? What is that likely to cost? What's the worst thing that can happen if I don't do what you recommend?" If the response to any or all of these queries is grim, seek another opinion. With a woman I know with a diagnosis similar to yours, the bad news was that she became somewhat incontinent, releasing a small amount of urine when she laughed, coughed or sneezed. The good news was that she suddenly became orgasmic during intercourse for the first time in her life. She felt that was more than adequate compensation for having to change panties several times a day and refused to consider having the condition fixed! In your case, I'd go back to the clinic or seek another and get some clarification first hand.

Is there some nice way to tell someone that you have no interest in going out with them socially?

There is the little white social lie: "My life is so very busy right now that I don't have time for a new friend." Or you might try the evasive truth: "Thank you for your invitation, but I'm sorry, I cannot." Only if someone persists might you feel the necessity of spelling out the fact that they personally are not what you are looking for as a friend. Whatever way you do choose (and please don't let it be a weasely "Not this time"; that only prolongs the discomfort for everybody), remember this person has paid you a compliment by seeking your company. A refusal accompanied by a return compliment ("I have enjoyed talking with you but....") and a kind touch, can soften the disappointing news.

The man I've been seeing for about three months always makes me be on top during sex. Always. After he comes he will not let me get off him until he wipes himself and me with a tissue which is always within arm's reach. It feels to me like he thinks sex is dirty. When I ask him about it, he simply doesn't answer. What do you think about this puzzling behavior?

I think your man has a strong case of "The Way It Has Gotta Be's." Asking him, or anyone for that matter, why he does what he does may get you *an* answer (although in your case it didn't), but rarely *the* answer—often because the person himself is unaware of the reasons. The best way around that is to make an observation rather than ask for an explanation. "I'm puzzled by your insistence on always having me on top. I'd like to be on the bottom for a change." You can open this conversation nonverbally, too, you know, by not getting on top or rolling onto your side, or leaping up before he gets a chance to wipe, or stopping his hand when he goes to wipe. You can even hide the ever-ready tissue box. Make some change in what usually happens, note his response, then use that as a jumping-off-place: "I notice that when I did this, you did that. I would like to understand you better. Would you be willing to talk about it?"

Much as I love my mate, there are times that I'm just not up for sex (or should I say "open to," since I am a woman?). Is there some way to say no without dire hurt feelings, particularly in the middle of the night when long explanations just aren't in order?

I don't know that long explanations for refusing sex are ever in order...but reassurance is: "I don't want to for reasons having to do with me rather than ones having to do with you." That's why "I have a headache" is more widely used than "You smell like a rutting goat." I have been lucky enough to know a lover who would take hold of my lasciviously questing hand under the covers, bring it to his lips for a kiss, and enfold it lovingly between his own and his pillow as he sank back into sleep. I'd be halfway to sleep again myself, a smile on my lips and a warm glow in my heart, before I realized that what he had just done was to say a nonverbal no to sex. But gee, the way he did it made me feel beloved and cherished—a sensation as good as, and probably better than, the one I originally sought.

I am a gay man who will soon be vacationing at a Club Med Resort, the mecca of heterosexuals worldwide. (Don't ask why I'm going, it's a long story.) Ever the optimist, I am sure there will be romantic opportunities even there if I go about this right. My problem is how do I go about uncovering such opportunities without getting punched in the snoot by some scandalized macho?

Ask Isadora

A dear friend of mine in a similar situation (a script writer, by the way) wrote what I think is a graceful and to-the-point line of dialogue for just such an occasion. "This is difficult to say (boyish grin), but I find myself attracted to you. If that's inappropriate, please take it as a compliment and we'll say no more about it. If not..." The ensuing pause is, dare I say it, "pregnant" with possibilities.

My husband simply will not talk about our sex life. He'll talk about sex in general like the rising incidence of sexually transmitted diseases, or he'll tell a joke with sexual content, but when I begin a discussion about what happens—or more often what does not happen—in our own bedroom, he'll do anything to avoid such a discussion, even pick a fight about the laundry. Is there any way you know of for me to engage him in some much-needed communication?

He has been communicating quite well, telling you in every way but in words that he does not want to discuss your sex life. I think it will enhance communication if you acknowledge that you have received his message: "You have made it perfectly clear that this is a discussion you would rather avoid, but I really need to insist." You could catch him where he quite literally cannot escape by bringing up the topic on a long drive, jumping into the shower stall with him, or perching on the tub rim while he's sitting on the commode. But I am much more in favor of seduction than psychological rape. Plan a picnic or a dinner at home with any children accounted for elsewhere and the phone unplugged. Rent a hot tub or a row boat on the lake. Make a date and create an uninterrupted time and place and then with all the love you can muster for this person who is obviously terrified of hearing bad news, tell him your satisfactions as well as your upsets. Be specific in what you want—more of this, less of that, and be sure to solicit his opinions on how you can assist in bringing about these desired changes.

I'm a modern woman. I even walk right into the drugstore in my own neighborhood to buy condoms. But when the time comes to introduce their use to a new partner who may balk, I turn into a timorous kid. What I want to do is shove the darn thing into his hand, mumble "Here," and disappear while he ponders it and, hopefully, puts it on. There are better ways, aren't there?

Most heavy issues are helped by a light touch. I have seen condoms marketed in the form of candy (right, condom mints), baked inside fortune cookies, sealed in clear boxes ("In case of emergency, break glass"), and wrapped in army camouflage ('Don't let them see you coming!"). The newest wrinkle in the "Yes, this is a serious business, but let's lighten up here, folks" approach is New Wave earrings, brooches and bolo ties made with glitzed-up condom packets. The sequins, glitter, feathers and paste jewels that adorn them do such a good job of discreetly veiling crass reality that even easy blushers could wear them out and about. Yet all this frou-frou does not damage the contents; underneath it all is a still-usable product. These things are usually a cottage industry product, (beats knitting toilet tissue roll covers), so look for them wherever you might find other adult novelties.

I am a 27-year-old gay man currently in a very happy relationship. Sometimes when I see a cute guy I think, "Hmm, I'd like to get into his pants." In the old days it seemed that's exactly what would happen. But what about nowadays? Is it normal to be in a relationship you're really happy with and still like looking at other guys? So far our relationship has been monogamous and I don't see any change in the future. But my community was once highly sexually charged and to a certain extent still is. Is there a way that I can tell people I think they're sexually appealing, but not have sex with them and not be labeled a P.T.? How do I deal with these feelings of attraction toward other guys?

The feelings you describe happen often in happy relationships of all denominations. The old line when admonished for being caught leering goes, "I'm married, not dead." Some people discharge lustful feelings for others in the conjugal bed overtly, spinning hot stories aloud for the titillation of both (often easier in same-sex relationships), or covertly, by fantasizing privately. If you and your partner trust yourselves and each other to keep within agreed-upon limits, I see nothing wrong in letting an attractive person know that "(sigh) if we had only met under different circumstances…" A P.T. keeps on promising what will not be delivered. The delight of consensual flirting is that two people get ego strokes and no one is hurt or disappointed.

At the age of 28, I recently had a breast augmentation. I'm perfectly happy with the results; that's not the problem. My sister, who has been the recipient of Nature's bounty since she was 12, thinks it necessary that everyone know (although if they care to look they can certainly see the change). What can I say to her to put the damper on such news bulletins as "Hey, have you seen my sister's new tits?" without hurting her feelings?

Somehow I doubt that she's as sensitive as you think her to be. How about a privately whispered and to the point statement: "Matilda (only if her name *is* Matilda!), I would prefer you not broadcast the fact of my operation." If she asks you how come, as some who know naught of subtlety may do, you need offer nothing more than "that's how I prefer it." Sometimes more than one application of this method is necessary, but keep at it until you achieve the desired silence.

chapter ten
Negotiating a Relationship

Ask Isadora

There seem to be mutually exclusive guidelines for satisfying others' needs and one's own. How can one experience sexual fulfillment without sacrificing one's personal freedom?

Which "one's"? I seem to be doing fine at the moment, so I deduce that it's you who's bucking some personal traffic. Behind the rhetoric what I think I'm hearing is "How can I play around when the person I love won't tolerate that?" Basically, it's a matter of negotiating a workable agreement. How about, "I love the time we spend together, and I need one (two, five) nights a week for myself." Whether you use that time to color your hair, read a good book, or to spend with other friends is your private business.

I am embarking on what feels like the greatest love affair of my life, and this time I want to make it work. Any suggestions?

Well, you might browse through a collection of happy homilies from couples married for 50 years ("Never go to bed angry," "Give in to the other person 75% of the time") and choose those that sound even remotely possible. But in my estimation, no one principle beats free-flowing honest communication, heavily seasoned with loving kindness, as the basis for a great ongoing relationship.

I've been dating, seeing, having an affair with, or whatever you want to call it, a man in his mid-30s for almost two years. Since he saw the replay of Annie Hall *on TV, he's been quoting Woody Allen's statement about relationships being like sharks who have to move forward or they die. I don't know what he wants to move forward to. I like things just as they are. Do you think it's true that relationships or people have to keep changing and growing? Can't someone or something just get where it should be and stay there?*

It sounds like what we're discussing here is some sort of "Peter Principle" of relationships. A favorite jump-rope rhyme when I was a little girl was "First comes love, then comes marriage, then comes you with a baby carriage." Unfortunately the myth still persists that relationships, or sex itself, must be like a Disneyland ride—once you take a ticket you've got to stay on and ride out a predetermined trip until the end; you can't get off until you get off, so to speak. These days, people can date (casually or exclusively), live together, marry, have a relationship that's monogamous or wide open, or any mutually agreeable variation on the theme. The operative words here are "mutually agreeable." Ask your lover what he wants to be different about the way you're spending time together; tell him what you like about the way things are, and negotiate from there. He might be caught up in some notion of "ought to" that, once examined, he'll discard with relief.

I've been seeing this man for the past year. Both of us have demanding, full-time jobs, so we don't see each other during the week. We've fallen into the pattern of spending our weekends together from Friday night to Sunday evening, sometimes at his apartment, sometimes at mine. The problem is that there are often social events on the weekends I'd like to go to, like parties given by friends, and he's not a very sociable fellow. So far, spending time with him has taken precedence, but I'm worried that if and when we break up, I'll have lost contact with everyone else I know and be really alone. How can I handle this?

What you're worried about is the wisdom of putting all your emotional eggs in one basket, and rightfully so. If attending the parties themselves is not an issue, perhaps you could maintain your other social contacts with occasional lunches, after-work cocktails, midweek early dinners, or post-dinner dessert dates. If you are missing the fun of *en masse* get-togethers, perhaps some halfway measure is possible—your lover accompanying you if you agree to stay a specified time only, your going alone on a Friday evening and joining him later, or going for a few hours on an occasional Saturday night if he declines to come with you. I think you are wise to give the arrangements you've fallen into a periodic reassessment. Even if you decide to make no changes, you can continue the relationship with renewed confirmation of your priorities.

A love affair that started several months ago when P. and I met has been what I've been looking for all my life. We haven't been apart since that first night except for our respective work and children. We're talking of getting married in the near future. This week, however, she spoke about missing the intensity of our initial time together. I'm trying not to be defensive, but realistically, how can a love affair continue to be as intense as it is when it first ignites? Isn't she mourning the impossible?

Wanting the impossible is not an uncommon state of affairs for romantics. Daniel Goldstine and co-authors in *The Dance-Away Lover*, and Susan Campbell in *The Couples' Journey*, among others, address the predictable stages in all love affairs. The time frame for each individual or couple may differ, but my own sense of the three-stage state of affairs goes like this: Stage I: "I'm absolutely enchanted by the way your nose wrinkles when you're amused". Stage II: "Don't twitch your nose at me, damn it. It's driving me bats." Stage III: "You have a unique way of smiling." Personally, I think Stage III is the good part. Sadly, it's also the part many people fail to hang in long enough to discover. It's when two people acknowledge each other, rather than their fantasies of each other—the good, the not-so-good, and the simple "what is." Check further into your lover's previous romantic history to see if she habitually loses interest after the initial hot-and-heavy. Also, try to get her to define precisely what she misses. (More lovemaking? Late night phone calls? Time spent with gazes locked?) See if it's something with which you are willing or able to keep her supplied.

I have fallen head over heels for a gay man. I'm female. He currently lives with another man with whom, he says, he's not too happy. He says he's tried relationships with women in the past, but he prefers men. Nonetheless, he says he's interested in trying again with me. I'm so attracted to him. Part of me wants to give it a try and another part says, "Forget it, he'll never change." Also I'd be concerned about AIDS. What do you think?

Let's start with the easiest part of your dilemma. The safe sex guidelines are quite clear and relate to any two people. You might want to know what precisely his sexual practices have been, how many partners he's had over the past five years or so, what precautions he's used, his health history and whether he's taken the AIDS antibody test and its results before deciding how physical to become. Whatever the facts, you can still hug, touch, and, depending on your own interpretation of what is safe, engage in intercourse using a condom. The issue of your *emotional* risk is another matter which depends a great deal on how each of you defines a "relationship." If your friend has strong erotic feelings toward men, that is extremely unlikely to change. His behavior, however, might. Some of the things you may need to look at together, as you would in entering into a relationship with any human being, is what your expectations are. Would you require sexual fidelity, for instance, or trust your partner to keep to any agreement you reach about emotional or sexual entanglements outside of those with you? If you can keep the lines of communication about your wants and needs honest and open, with yourself as well as with him, your relationship, whatever its form, can be a good one. I have had and continue to have several deeply satisfying relationships with bisexual and gay men, some of which have included sexual activity, all of which include sexual feelings. I wouldn't have missed any of them for any price...including the occasional grieving for what could not be.

I am a 25-year-old woman. Last winter I got involved in an intimate relationship with a man my age. After a few months we saw that it wasn't working out so we decided to remain friends and see other people. We're still attracted to each other and are often physically affectionate, though no longer sexually involved. Recently he acquired a new housemate whom I find very attractive. I'm reluctant to discuss my interest in his housemate with my friend. He's a bit sensitive and once indicated that he didn't want to hear about other involvements on my part. (I don't hear about his either). Would it be tasteless of me to let the housemate know I'm interested and how could I do this tactfully without damaging any of the friendships involved?

It's anybody's guess whether such a transition can be accomplished without hurt feelings on somebody's part, but let's explore some ways to minimize that risk. If the two men "hang out" together, either at home or outside, hang out with them. Within this camaraderie you can get to know the housemate better and assess the likelihood of mutual interest. If there's none, why upset your friend? Or, consider "bumping into" the housemate when he's alone and assessing the chances after that meeting. Another suggestion is to have a hypothetical discussion with your friend: "If I were attracted to a friend of yours, how would you prefer I handle it?" All of these are suggestions on ways to hedge your bets from one who usually opts for straight-out honesty. But I can't really see the wisdom of risking your friendship by a premature declaration of intent if nothing will come of it.

My wife is a lovely woman with a classic hourglass figure any woman would envy. How can I get her to throw off her inhibitions and be unashamed to be naked in my presence? As it is now, she goes out of her way to make sure that I don't see her unclothed.

How you can get her to throw off her inhibitions when she won't even throw off her clothes is beyond me. You may be expecting too much of a change, and too quickly at that. Tell her how you feel: "I feel left out when you undress behind closed doors," or "I really would enjoy seeing you nude more often. Is there any way I could help you feel more comfortable doing that?" Stating your feelings and wishes in this manner, rather than in the accusatory "Why don't you...?", may encourage her to explain hers. Then together you might negotiate something between abandon and prudery which would be comfortable for both.

Ask Isadora

While my problem is not with "an intimate," my relationship with the woman with whom I share a two-person office is certainly an intimate one in that I spend more of my waking hours alone with her than I do with my wife, child, or any of my chosen friends. I enjoy my work itself, but just the thought of having to face her each morning—her gum chewing, her nail tapping, her inane attempts at social conversation, fills me with dread and spoils the day before it begins. What can I do, or at least, where can I begin?

I have an Ashleigh Brilliant "Pot Shot" postcard framed on the wall of my counseling office. It states: "If you can't go around it, over it, or through it, you had better negotiate with it." If you have already tried the obvious arounds, overs and throughs of securing a private office, keeping different hours, working at home, etc, then all that's left, other than leaving or continuing on as things are until you explode, is negotiating. Take the most obvious irritation and begin with it, framing your dilemma without blame and perhaps with a stroke or two in her direction: "I know it must get boring for you without any conversation, but I really have to concentrate on what I'm doing in order to get anything done at all. If I don't respond when you ask me something, put it down to my compulsive work habits." That's not a "You're a pain" message, but an "I'm the pill" one. Nonetheless, you have put her on notice that you won't respond to her distractions. Then don't. One by one, you may be able to lessen the irritants in this way. When you've succeeded, you may be able to really see this woman and her needs and willingly provide some of the attention, respect, or whatever she may be seeking, not out of magnanimity, but out of self-preservation.

Isadora Alman

The new woman in my life is a very sexy lady, except for one thing. She does not shave under her arms. I know that shaving or not is a matter of taste, but it really turns me off. I told her how I feel and her response was "They're my armpits." Now what?

A compromise with one shaven and one un? Nah, I guess not. At first blush the issue does appear to be a matter of personal taste, but superseding that seems to be a power struggle fairly typical to new couples over who's more willing to accommodate whom. Perhaps you might bring the contest of wills into the open by staging a spelling bee or a thumb wrestling match, or shaving your own pits, seeing what she has to say about that, and negotiating from there.

I'm 18 years old and have been in a lock-down institution for the past eight months. I have a girlfriend on the outside who says she loves me and will wait for me. Then she tells me she wants to go out with another guy. When I try to talk to her and tell her how I feel she tells me I only call to argue and that it's none of my affair. I don't know what to do.

There isn't much you can do. If she won't listen to what you have to say on the phone, try writing her a letter. Eighteen is awfully young to make or expect a commitment, no matter how great your need. I realize that this won't be much of a comfort to you, but even if you were not in prison, the situation would look the same. A person is going to do what they're going to do regardless of the "righteousness" of your arguments.

I am in a terrific, very sensual and sexual relationship with a great man. Everything is working well and it looks long term. There's only one minor glitch, and I'm not sure if I'm just not being overly

Ask Isadora

sensitive. My lover is horny for me practically daily, or even more, but he also masturbates regularly. It's not as if he stops paying attention to me. He says he just masturbates because he likes it. In fact, he has been known to do so several times a day even on days we make love. My problem? I think I'm jealous of him playing with himself. It's as if jacking off is as much fun and as important as making love to me. Should I just stop worrying about this or what?

Even if, on a secret satisfaction scale of 1 to 10, he assigned jacking off a higher rating than making love to you, what could you do about it? His masturbating doesn't seem to affect desire for or sex with you. Presumably he's not likely to abandon these practices, so should you stop worrying about this or what? When given a choice, I'd go for no worry over worry every time.

I'm always looking for new ways to put some zing in my marriage of almost twenty-five years. Whenever I suggest something even a little bit sexy like going to a private hot tub place or trying out some mentholated massage oil, my husband's response is usually, "C'mon, we're too old for that kind of stuff." What do you think, Isadora? Is there some particular age when a person is too old to try out new and potentially pleasurable things?

Yes, posthumously. Until and right up to that point, of course not. My response to your husband would be, "What do you mean *we're* too old, Grandpa?" What he seems to be telling you is that he is feeling old. You might suggest a physical checkup, some reading on ageing bodies and minds, and frequent reassurances that you still find him a desirable playmate—no pressure to perform, only to come on out and play.

My boyfriend and my closest woman friend seem to have eyes for each other. Rather than lose either of them, is there some way I or we could combine our relationships?

The French have a name for what you are proposing and it has a time-honored tradition—a *ménage à trois*, a three-way arrangement. Such arrangements can work in several ways—one pivotal person relating sexually to each of the others with everyone's knowledge and consent, or, for all three to relate sexually to each other. What distinguishes a ménage à trois from one person with two separate lovers is that all people involved in it have emotional and affectionate ties, and the relationship(s) is usually ongoing. Before upping the ante in your own, may I suggest a private heart-to-heart talk with each of your dear ones, sounding them out on the idea and stating your own fantasies and fears. I'm not saying the risk may not be worth it, but with something this hot someone could get burned.

On your radio show you advised a woman who was apprehensive about getting back into dating that she had no obligation "to lift her skirt" in appreciation to the man who wines and dines her. Quite right, absolutely. However, consider that the dating ritual is a mating ritual. If a woman wines and dines a man, he also puts himself in some degree of assumed or implied obligation. (But neither should he be obliged to lift his kilt in appreciation!) The moral: A "suitee" who does not want to be compromised might be well advised to insist on paying half the evening's expenses. What about it, Isadora?

I do agree that insistence on paying one's own way is the best insurance against the creep who views dating as a covert prostitution negotiation: "Let's see, I spent $45 on dinner, $12 on movie tickets, so you owe me three sloppy kisses and a hand job." But that's not all an invitation out for an evening is about, is it? While dating may equal courtship with an aim in view, as you imply (getting the other person to...commit, screw, marry, whatever), it can also be a mutual exploration of the possibilities between you two (Can we be friends, lovers, can I sell you some real estate?). As such, the one to play host first is usually the one with the keenest interest or strongest agenda, the one assumed to have the most discretionary income, or the one with the social moxie to make the first move. Fortunately or un, by all those criteria it is usually the male.

A young lady and I have been enjoying a good sexual relationship for the past few months. She has been cooperative in every way except on the matter of oral sex. She has said that she does not want to taste my emissions, and even though I have assured her I will take care not to ejaculate, we have argued over this without any satisfactory conclusion. Because of our differences she has also refused cunnilingus. I believe that our relationship can be enhanced if I have some reference material which I can use to convince her that oral activities are a vital part of sex play just as much as the fingering she enjoys prior to intercourse. Any assistance in finding books that treat on this matter will be appreciated.

I intended to respond that any good book on general sexuality would have something to say on the subject, but in checking in my own library I find to my surprise that it isn't so. Such basics as Alex Comfort's *The Joy of Sex,* and Helen Singer Kaplan's *Making Sense of Sex,* omit any mention of oral sex. In *Making Love* (New York, Dial Press: 272 pps., $14.95. Avon paperback, $8.95), which is subtitled *The Most Thorough &*

Explicit Guide to Sexual Fulfillment Ever Published, Patricia E. Raley writes: "Kinsey found that the longer people were together or the more experienced they were, the more likely they were to try to enjoy oral sex. But many people saw it then and see it now as a perversion....Although the laws against oral sex aren't invoked very often, they do reinforce the notion that there is something inherently evil about a very widespread practice." Following a sample dialogue between a man who wants oral sex, with his arguments pro, and his female partner who doesn't, and her arguments con, the author writes: "The symbolic issues of dominance and subservience may lie behind the praise of sensations or the complaint about smell, but it is easiest to deal directly with the physical aspects first. Sometimes this is the best way to reach the symbolic issues as well." The author then goes on to give some excellent practical suggestions on gentle education of a reluctant partner of either sex.

What this book, published in 1976, does not address is the present-day caution against oral contact with body emissions. (No matter what you promise, you really cannot be sure!) Your woman friend's objections may come, not from ignorance of the joys of oral sex, but awareness of its possible dangers. In that case, using a condom on you and a dental dam on her may be your solution.

Romance in my relationship of many years seems to have died. Sex is fine while we're having it, but leading up to it is always coarse and abrupt and two minutes after it's over he's talking about the Giants, our finances, or current events again. So far I've tried being more romantic myself (which he ridicules), talking about it gently (which he treats as

Ask Isadora

torture), making myself more attractive (which he doesn't notice), and varying the daily routine with more inspired activities (which he resists or refuses). I'm still crazy about him, but I'm too young to kiss off lingering kisses and the wide open spaces of romantic sex. Should I give up?

If you're comparing a relationship of many years to an initial courtship, practically anyone's is bound to suffer in such areas as seductively-served dinners, soul-baring conversations which last until dawn, and inarticulate declarations of passionate desire. (I think love affairs which have had some mellowing time have different, often better plusses, but many people disagree.) Think clearly now, was this beloved lout of yours *ever* really romantic in your terms? You write that romance has died, as if it once lived, but it sounds to me that you are asking someone who is totally colorblind to select your favorite tint of mauve. Spell out the behaviors you want in exquisite detail just as if you were paper-training a puppy and, as with the puppy, lavishly reward anything which even gets close to the mark. ("Hey, this time you stayed in bed for a full five minutes before getting up and turning on the ball game. Thank you, I really enjoyed the extra cuddling.") There is no need to quit hoping or trying *if* you regard your attempts with rueful amusement rather than growing frustration and bitterness. If the latter, spare yourself the sweat you work up by beating a dead horse and seek your romance RDA via extracurricular flirtations or Barbara Cartland novels.

The woman I have been seeing for several months has had a job transfer to another state; she's leaving within the month. We're both in our 30s and confirmed the fact early on in our dating that each of us was looking for a long-term mate with whom to raise a family. Obviously we each see the other as a distinct possibility in this role, but it's just too soon to make a commitment, for me at least, and, I suspect, for her, too. The imminence of her departure, however, makes me feel that we have to make some decision before she goes—to become engaged, to break it off, whatever. How do I handle this when I don't feel ready to do either?

With what I usually recommend—honest communication, with yourself first and then with her. It sounds like you know what you feel and what you want—more time together to make an enlightened choice. Since you don't mention her pushing for some commitment or some input on whether or not to take this transfer, it sounds like the necessity to decide now is a self-imposed "should" which can just as easily be self-unimposed. Talk to her. Tell her honestly how you feel and what you want. If she also is undecided on commitment yet is not willing to end it, work something out. Discuss your fears and hopes about monogamy arrangements, letters, phone calls, holiday visits, etc. And at least agree to rediscuss your mutual feelings sometime in the near future, perhaps planning a visit together in three to six months. Continuing an exploratory courtship via long distance is not impossible, just damnably difficult. You get to decide, having tried it out, whether it's worth it.

My husband of thirteen years and I divorced about eighteen months ago. I've seen other people, he's seen other people, and we continue to see each other occasionally. When we do, we usually have sex. I admit I haven't found anyone as interesting to me as he is, yet the reasons our marriage dissolved (differences about money, career, values) are still as true today as they were before. He wants us to either recommit or break off, saying this relationship is neither fish nor fowl. I don't want to marry this man again and I certainly can't imagine us being strangers. Isn't there something else?

Of course there is. Look at all the people in your life. The relationship you have with A isn't exactly like the relationship you have with B, even if both might be female friends, or cousins, or co-workers. Perhaps your husband can't conceive of any possibilities other than spouse or stranger, but now that you have, try to sell him on the idea—defining and refining until you negotiate something that feels okay to both of you at the moment.

I am a woman who loves sexual intercourse. If my lover tapped me on the shoulder when I was cleaning the fish bowl I would be ready before he got his pants unbuckled. And I would be finished, including a satisfying orgasm, within 90 seconds. Every quick-coming man's dream, right? The problem is my lover, a New Age sensitive type, was trained by some other woman or women to not begin the main event without at least a half-hour of preliminaries. No matter how I try to rush things along to the "good" part, he keeps holding himself back in what I imagine he imagines is a gentlemanly manner. He doesn't seem to get that it just isn't necessary with me. What now?

There is the possibility that what you call preliminaries are necessary for *him*. Just as you give the lie to the myth that all woman need lots of pre-intercourse warm-up, there are many men who are *not* ready, willing and instantly able at the drop of a hint. At some non-sexual time, tell him in plain words how much you like "quickies" and that it would turn you on for him to act upon his urges sometimes. If that is just not physically or psychologically his style, you may just have to accept it. I know a woman who is the kind of avid sports nut who would go to a stadium in a blizzard for a marbles tournament. She fell in love with a man who doesn't know a football from a hockey puck and has no interest in learning. Cupid often has a weird sense of humor when he shoots those darts.

Reader response: I wonder if the lady has tried making use of the erections which her lover probably has during his REM sleep. Before I learned of normal erections during REM sleep I heard a man tell of waking from an erotic dream and finding his wife impaled on his penis and nearing her orgasm. I could not imagine my (hence, his) being able to sleep through the exquisite sensation accompanying insertion, but perhaps that sensation served to direct or modify the path his dream took. Wild guess/hope: Maybe the dreaming could fool his psyche into believing that the "preliminaries" were already over. That way he could proceed or continue since she had already taken the initiative with his REM sleep-induced erection.

I'll give your suggestion some thought. Let's sleep on it.

I guess I'm one of your younger readers. I'm 17. I have a girlfriend my age who is also a virgin. She wants to have sex with me. I don't want to. What do I do?

Nancy Reagan not only gave you her personal support, she told you loudly and often just what to tell your girlfriend: "Just say no." I'm sure you would be able to do that if she asked you to participate in some other activity that you don't care to try, right? The belief that

Ask Isadora

all red-blooded men will jump at any occasion to have any kind of sex is absurd. You might, if she is a friend you can really level with, tell her some of your reasons for refusing. (You don't feel ready, you're afraid of the risk, she doesn't attract you in that way, you prefer to wait for love or marriage.) I want to assure you that you don't owe her any explanations, but in the name of kindness, if not of friendship, you do owe her tactful gentleness. So "No, thank you," plus some reassurances about her attractiveness, or your willingness to continue the friendship are definitely in order.

How do you know when someone is stringing you along, and what can be done about it? This woman says she loves me, but she also says this relationship won't work and we'd better end it while we're ahead. Does that make sense to you?

The operative question here is what do you *want* to do. That cuts right through the "what's going on here?" and the "shoulds." Emotions rarely do make "sense." That's why they are feelings and not facts. It is possible that she may both love you and also wish to end the relationship—she may not love you "enough" by her lights or yours, may also love someone or something more, may have a different life plan than yours. All those possibilities might account for the hot and cold actions which could well feel to you like being strung along. If she can't explain or you can't understand any better than you have, then back to the basic choice. It's painful being with her right now and will probably be painful without her for a while. Choose the one you feel you can handle best or is likely to lead where you want to go.

A popular song speaks of someone wanting to hear soothing lies from her lover instead of the truth. My impression is that most partners and prospective partners in intimate relationships want emotional reassurances, and in such an atmosphere people come to expect lies instead of truthfulness. I don't think it's lack of communication skills, but rather bending the truth to satisfy the other person's expectations. I'm sure you have some editorial remarks, but I would really like to know of any good studies on honesty in relationships.

I think what you are discussing *is* communication skills. The clarification of expectations and the making of agreements to be honest with each other (or not to be, if the truth is too painful) is a necessary part of forming an intimate relationship. Any good book on creating or maintaining intimate relationships will address these issues. A few of my favorites are Susan Campbell's *The Couples' Journey*, Bach and Deutsch's *Pairing: How to Achieve Genuine Intimacy*, and *Lovestyles: How to Celebrate Your Differences* by Tina Tessina. For specific, professional experimental studies you will need to check the abstracts of psychology, communication and marital relations journals in any good library.

In a year and a half of living together my previous girlfriend probably had three orgasms through simple intercourse. In the past four years my present girlfriend hasn't had one three times. She'll have her first one within a minute or two of penetration and will frequently have a second and occasionally a third before I reach my one and only. I'd like to think of myself as giving her orgasms, but in fact, she takes them from me. A guy gets to feeling used. Are there any techniques I can use to restore the more natural 90:10 man/woman power balance? Just once I'd like to feel as though I've deprived her of an orgasm. Am I sick?

Sick? I wouldn't choose that word; it's so pejorative. How about "nasty"?

I am a 32-year-old-man with a 29-year-old-female partner. My problem is that I cannot seem to accept the idea of a monogamous relationship. How do I carry on relations with a woman without getting involved in a confining, sexually exclusive relationship? And how do I tell my current amour that I am unsure about carrying on our monogamous relationship of more than a year without hurting her terribly?

One possibility is to cheat. That solution has the advantage of having a long and time-honored history. Negotiating an open relationship is not easy, and in some cases it isn't possible, but in more cases than you think, it is. So if ethics forbid lying (as I hope they do), check out J. Smith and L. Smith's collection of essays, *Beyond Monogamy,* Ronald Mazur's *The New Intimacy: Open-Ended Marriage and Alternative Lifestyes,* or *How To Be A Couple And Still Be Free,* by Tessina & Smith. Then gird your loins and tell your lover that the two of you need to talk.

I have known this very nice girl for more than a year now. We're good friends and get along very well. I have been accustomed to treating her like the rest of my friends, but now my feelings have betrayed me. I would like to become more than an ordinary friend and get more personally involved with her, but I don't know how to approach her. What would she think if I disclose my feelings? If she does not feel the same way that I feel, I might lose her friendship and I really don't want that to happen.

And if she does share your feelings, think how delightful the love affair might be and how happy you would feel to have taken the risk. That's what risk is about—the possibility of a loss is offset by the possibility of an equal, or greater, "win." If the loss seems worse to you than the potential pay-off, then the risk is too great. In this case you might hedge your bet a bit by some abstract communication ("Do you think it's possible that two people who start out as friends could ever be more to each other than that?"). If she does not think such a scenario is possible, you have a fairly good idea of her feelings for you without personal disclosure. In the case of testing for romantic or sexual feelings, however, I'm in favor of non-verbal investigations. Prolong your customary goodnight hug, take her hand in a playful fashion during a movie, offer to exchange backrubs. See what happens when you touch. If there's sizzle potential there, it can often get through where words might only get in the way.

I am the type of person who likes to have sex for a long time, not just fifteen or twenty minutes. My boyfriend just seems to get really tired after he comes. I also like to have sex more than once a week and he doesn't. What should I do?

How about beating him with a used condom until he conforms to your desires? Seriously, what *can* you do? You are dealing with a fellow human being here and his capabilities and preferences in this most personal of self-expressions. Tell him your preferences and see what you two can come up with that will allow you to have at least some of your preferences some of the time. For instance, maybe he would be willing to occasionally take a long, slow time in pleasing you in other ways than intercourse and then enjoy his own pleasure in his preferred manner. If by any chance you intend "having sex for a long time" to mean having intercourse (some people do equate the two), you really can't expect a man to last more than five minutes or so. Though some do by nature or training, the average length of intercourse in our culture is less than three minutes. Also, though some men have other patterns, it is quite usual to be tired after an orgasm since what an orgasm is is a release of tension. As for wanting more sex than your partner does, by redefining "sex" to include cuddling or mutual caressing or reading erotic books together—non-intercourse activities that encourage closeness—the two of you might bring your desires more into alignment.

I am a single parent who has raised a daughter alone since the age of 2. She is now 13. She seems less and less willing to do the things we've always done together, preferring the company of her friends or even being alone in her room to being with me. For example, Sunday afternoon we were on the way out to the movies when she got a phone call from a friend inviting her elsewhere. She accepted eagerly. I felt abandoned. How can I get her to see the selfishness of such behavior?

Um, Mom (or Dad, as the case may be), since you asked, I must say that I don't think it's your daughter who is being the selfish one here. Rude and a bit thoughtless, perhaps, but for an adolescent to prefer the company of her peers to that of a parent is natural and healthy. For an adult to continue to seek the company of an adolescent rather than his or her peers is not. By all means speak with your daughter about keeping commitments to you and to others, but try to muster the good grace to support her emerging independence and begin to broaden your own social network.

Isadora Alman

I am a man who is fed up with the way so many women nowadays insist on men using condoms. I don't care what anyone says, they do reduce the pleasure, and I find them a barrier to real intimacy. My question is this: Suppose I put on a condom (because the woman insisted) and then, just before penetration, took it off without her noticing. Is there any way she could tell during intercourse that I wasn't still wearing it?

Let us suppose that a former lover, one with whom you felt you had a satisfying intimate relationship, showed up at your door this afternoon, handed you a shrieking infant and said, "Here. I know I told you I was taking birth control pills when we were sexual together, but I lied. I became pregnant, had the baby, and now he's your responsibility." No matter how you feel about being a parent, don't you think you might, at best, be taken aback by such an abrupt revelation, maybe experience even stronger feelings—not all of them pleasant? While a woman might not be able to tell if you were wearing a condom during intercourse, might not even be able to tell upon ejaculation, the message about what kind of man you are would be unequivocally communicated. So if you think a teensy thickness of latex is a "barrier to intimacy," I assure you that a "Hah hah, I fooled you!" approach to putting a partner at risk for an unwanted pregnancy, let alone disease, is not an improvement. I suggest you look anew at your definition of intimacy. It is not a synonym for screwing...or getting screwed.

chapter eleven
Exotica

Ask Isadora

I'm a guy, 22, and I live with my folks. My sister just returned home after a bad marriage. One night, when we were both stoned, she had me dress up in her clothes and I really got off on it. I suggested doing it again several times, but I guess she lost interest. I haven't. What do you think about my dressing in her clothes when she's not home?

We have two issues here. One is a matter of manners. I don't think it's ever appropriate for people who share living quarters to use each other's personal belongings without prior consent. I can see where making that arrangement might be more of a confrontation with your sister than you might want to have. The other issue is about cross-dressing in general, which I think is what you're asking me about. Dressing in women's clothes, or some particular items of them, is highly erotic for certain men. Some choose to do this with their partners and turn the event into a sexy little drama interesting to both parties. You don't mention an erotic play partner (other than your sister, which is not a great idea at your age). Many men do use women's clothing as part of solitary sexual fantasy. If this is something you want to explore further, it's not a big investment to buy the necessaries for yourself at a thrift shop or garage sale. One word of caution—high heels can be a bitch.

This summer I intend to go to a nude beach for the first time. I guess the idea is the same—lots of naked people hanging out and having fun. What's the scoop? What should I know so that I won't embarrass myself?

One convention that will stand you in good stead is eye contact, lots of eye contact. Every man I've ever spoken to who was about to be nude in mixed company for the first time had two main fears. One is that he might get an erection, and the other is that he might not. If you decide ahead of time that either possibility will be okay with you, and that your intention is to have a good time, you will.

I inherited a cat about two years old from a male neighbor who moved away. I don't know a lot about cats, but Blackie and I seem to be getting along. I've noted that although the cat doesn't seem to be altered, he shows no interest in the cries of neighborhood female cats, but shows a remarkably keen interest in my male visitors. Is it possible for a cat to be gay? Is this an "only in San Francisco" question?

You've heard of bestiality—human sexual contact with animals? Your Blackie may be a practitioner of "humanality," preferring cross-species contact from his own perspective. He may also miss his former owner on whom he may have imprinted as a parent figure. He may be altered (your cat, not your former neighbor). A vet visit would be helpful in determining that. Finally, yes, cats and all other animals may be gay, in the sense of enjoying sexual behavior with same-sex members of their own species—everywhere, not only in San Francisco.

Is there anything actually dangerous in being sexy with my dog? I mean, can I catch some disgusting disease or something?

Dogs can and have been trained to do all kinds of tricks more interesting than rolling over and playing dead. You could, if you're male, wear a condom. I don't know about fitting one on a dog. Dogs' penises have some unique properties, especially during intercourse, so if you are thinking along those lines, be sure to read up on their physiology. Other than that, there are fleas, poison oak from their coats, or bites and scratches which would be a dog's way of saying, "Not tonight, dear. I have a headache."

Reader response #1: *Recently your column featured a letter from someone who wanted to know if it could be dangerous to be "sexy" with her/his dog. Two weeks later several letters to the editor protested your answer on the grounds that it condoned cruelty to animals. I'm inclined to agree. It seems to me that animals rank along with children in that they are unable to give their consent to sexual acts. I'd appreciate your comments on this.*

Response #2: *You advocated the use of animals for human sexual gratification without giving any consideration to the tremendous inequality which exists between people and their pets. Most dogs won't growl at or bite their owners no matter what they do to them.*

I'm quoting from the above letters because they do raise an important point and they do so in a rational manner. (Though I did love the letter from the man who suggested that I take "a standard size condom, one suitable for use on dogs, perhaps," and pull it over my head.) I do not advocate sex acts with animals. I do not advocate any kind of sexual behavior. I simply inform as a sex educator or opine as a columnist, and try always to make a distinction between the two. I have advocated, nay, actively championed the concept of informed, mutual consent in any social or sexual interaction. I thought I had dealt with consent, albeit flippantly, by demonstrating that an animal declines consent by biting, scratching, or simply walking away in disinterest. The letter writer did not identify him or herself as male or female, nor as the potential initiator or recipient of the dog's sexual attentions. If you've ever had your crotch sniffed, leg humped, or petting hand directed genital-ward by a wriggling dog in rut, you'll realize that animals are often the sexual aggressors. Whether the human chooses to ignore such behavior, to train the animal not to do these "natural" animal acts, to neuter the creature or have it mated, or to accommodate it-, him-, or herself, is a matter of personal situational ethics. I can see, however, that for many people perceived power abuse is at issue here, inherent in the owner/animal relationship in the same way dependency issues affect the concept of spousal rape or defining a legal age of consent. It is a valid point and I appreciate the manner in which these writers brought it to my attention.

I just moved to a neighborhood where the view is 90% of what I'm paying for in rent. To enjoy it more, I bought a pair of binoculars and I'm getting views that city planners did not intend to provide. Twice I've seen couples making love in unshaded windows and for the past week there has been an eruption of unselfconscious masturbators. I'm not sure whether I have inadvertently stumbled upon some local version of Show and Tell or what. Am I supposed to reciprocate? Can you enlighten me?

Some localities have a custom of calling at the door of newcomers to introduce the neighbors. Welcome to Fun City. San Francisco isn't called The City That Knows How for nothing. As for whether or not you're expected to return the courtesy, perhaps you might ask Miss Manners.

I don't want to get disgustingly graphic, but there's no way to put this delicately. Some of my office friends were talking about a story one of them actually read in a newspaper about somebody inserting a gerbil into his anus for some sort of way-out kicks. Is that possible?—not that somebody did something nefariously sexual with a small animal—I'm well aware of the unbounded stretches of the creative human mind—but that such a story was printed somewhere?

Will the animal rights activists who are reeling in shock from the question please skip the next part? I have already heard, and sympathized, with the views of many of you, but I'm still going to answer the question. A story on this topic did indeed appear in the press. (It was not one of the supermarket-type tabloids. The doer of the deed would have had to have had a subsequent religious revelation for it to merit their attention.) Knowing my penchant for reading sexual and relationship-oriented oddities on the first part of my radio show, a listener sent me a clipping from an East Coast newspaper. It was a Q and A column written by a man who promises to trace to their source answers to all sorts of oddball queries. Alas, I didn't keep the clipping (or read it on the air), but it concerned tracking the meaning of "gerbil sex." The idea was that a supposedly de-clawed little critter was induced somehow to crawl into someone's bodily orifice for the fantasized pleasurable sensations its maneuvers would cause. Supposedly, the beastie died in the process, and the creative genius who thought up the idea had to go to a hospital emergency room to have its carcass removed. I would love to have been there to hear his explanation. Any of you who have intimates who work in hospitals will have heard stories of people who "just happened to have sat on a cucumber" or "inexplicably" got their penis caught in the hose while they were vacuuming naked. And no, to forestall any further questions, I earnestly doubt there might be any pleasurable sensations involved in such an experiment—not for the anus owner, and certainly not for the gerbil.

What has spanking got to do with sex? How can it possibly be pleasurable? Can it be politically correct? The reason I ask is that it turns me on, particularly as spanker but also as spankee. It has also been a real turn-on for several, though not all, of my lovers. Most of the time the subject of spanking, even when raised in the abstract, leads to an uncomfortable rebuke. Obviously, I never force it on anyone. Just as obviously, this periodic need of mine often goes unfulfilled. So what can I do? I feel that your usual position of accepting all consenting sexuality needs a bit of clarification for this one. After all, spanking is not just another way of rubbing a loved one in a special way. I feel that feminism must be taken into account, particularly in light of the potential for violence against women. And spanking as pleasure must be explained when faced with the obvious fact that it often, although not always, hurts. Since I've tried for years to figure all of this out, I would sure appreciate the benefit of your insight.

I don't know what all-encompassing polemic I can offer. You're right, 'tis a puzzlement that pain (or humiliation) can sometimes be a pleasurable exchange *when consensual*. Psychotherapy is one avenue of exploration if you really want to understand its import to you personally. Otherwise, since you are able to find occasional partners who are willing to play in your arena, you might as well relax and enjoy those juicy discussions of ethical pros and cons and personal predilections which uncover kindred souls.

Ask Isadora

A gay friend of mine introduced me (verbally) to the marvels of safe sex orgies by recounting his experiences at a private j.o. club. Except for the lack of females present, it sounded great to me. Is there such a place for heterosexuals?

Privately there is. A group in San Francisco called Mother Goose Productions gives monthly by-invitation-only parties called Jack and Jill-Offs open to ones, twos and threes of all persuasions—not just gays, not only straights. Behaviors vary, making and watching erotic videos, verbal fantasy exchanges, body rubbing, masturbation, and watching and being watched, all without any contact with body fluids. The rules: "No fucking, no unprotected oral action, no poppers, no rude behavior, ask before touching." If it's happening in San Francisco, can Anytown, USA be far behind?

My current lover says he's heard that strangling a man when he comes gives him a practically subatomic climax. It has something to do with cutting off the oxygen or blood flow to the brain. Do you have any tips on how to do this without any undesirable complications...such as killing him?

My tip is: DON'T TRY IT! You are risking hemorrhage, stroke, brain damage and death when you naively aim for "just the right amount" of strangulation. I am convinced that a large percentage of what looks like suicides by hanging are really masturbatory experiments which failed, particularly among teenage males. The consequences of their curiosity turned out to be far more tragic than a botched orgasm.

After reviewing some books you suggested on oral sex, my partner and I arrived at a clearer under-

standing about oral sex and its potential erotic value. We both agreed to engage in it this past weekend and the results were excellent. Now that her sexual awareness and arousal has been broadened, do you think she should be gifted with a dildo also?

Some women prefer flowers or perfume, but sure, why not? A gift of a sexual toy needs to be looked at in just that way, as a toy to play with if it so pleases. No "shoulds," no hidden messages. If she doesn't find it erotic or amusing, it says nothing about the "width" of her newly broadened sexual awareness, just her own personal preference.

My friend and lover recently expressed a fantasy of having two women making love to him at once—together, taking turns, in combinations, and so forth—not necessarily to each other. I'm willing, but neither of us can figure out how to recruit the other woman! He's not currently dating anyone else. I have tentatively brought the subject up to several of my woman friends but no one has nibbled at the bait. He lives out-of-state, so the idea of starting to include a friend in our activities in order to let her get to know him well just isn't practical. He seems to prefer that I do the arranging. He's suggested a romantic dinner for three at my place that would hopefully segue into the bedroom. But it seems to me I'd have to give the other woman a hint of what was planned in order for it to work. Have you any recommendations on how to get this accomplished?

I've seen a few personal ads in respectable papers lately seeking friendships likely to lead to the same arrangement; or there are sexually explicit publications which carry ads. Think of cruising groups or events, such as swing party houses or alternative lifestyle associations which attract the sexually adventurous. Wherever or whenever you find a likely candidate, I feel it's necessary to do more than hint at your hopes. If you are willing to be a bit bolder with the women you do know and just say, as you did to me, "We'd like this but not that," you might not have to go to the trouble, expense (and possibly the fun) of a search among strangers.

I don't know whether to address this question to you or the guy who writes the veterinary column in the Chronicle. *Somehow, I think I'll get a more direct answer from you. My question is: How big is an elephant's penis?*

I quote from a marvelous book by Robert A. Wallace called *How They Do It* (N.Y: Morrow & Co., 1980, $4.95): "...about four or five feet long...at full erection...a peculiar S-shape, and the end swells into an enormous bulb." If that isn't enough to plunk your twanger, read on: "...the penis does the positioning. It moves, snakelike, up and down and from side to side, searching for the vaginal opening. When his search has been successful...his penis vigorously jerks up and down, probing at the vagina again and again until it enters her." Throughout all this, I presume the male elephant is still attached to—if not in control of—this amazing appendage!

I've usually cast a scant eye toward your column from the days of your anal/gerbil advice. But after your recent column I will be a devoted reader and pledge allegiance to Isadora if I can only discover some way, just for one night, to have my nipples tortured by an elephant's penis.

I do not make up the letters I print, I swear it!

Isadora Alman

When we broke up, my last lover bought me a vibrator and I don't know whether to thank him or curse him. All the great feelings of being with a man and having him caress and fondle me cannot be replaced by the vibrator, but I need one in order to have an orgasm. I hate it! I wish I'd learned to have orgasms manually. I have tried to wean myself from using it, but I either get bored, or lose the orgasm, or get so worked up that I give in and use the vibrator to take me over the edge. How can I make the switch in masturbation and how can I tell a sex partner that I need a vibrator to come? Will a man understand and not feel threatened?

Some men do feel threatened, some understand, and some are both relieved at not having the full responsibility for your climax and turned on as well by watching you do it on your own. You can't know how it will be until it is. One method is to incorporate both: "I'd like to come with you holding me in your arms while I use my vibrator. How would that be?" As for making the switch on your own, it can be done eventually, but why struggle so? Some of your masturbation can be a learning or training ground, sure, but if self-pleasuring ceases to become that, where oh where can a person turn? *Play* with fingers, play with water, play with different kinds of vibrators and different kinds of fantasies. If you develop as broad a range of what gets you off as possible, you can, on any given occasion, *choose* your *preferred* method rather than resort to your *only*.

I'm a 26-year-old lesbian, and after years of playing with my vibrator and its attachments I thought I'd go for the next step up and try a dildo. So I went off to my friendly neighborhood sex toy store and bought one. When I got my new toy home I was disappointed to find I simply couldn't get the damn

Ask Isadora

thing in. It's been four or five years since I had sex with a man and I can't remember exactly how big erect penises are, but this thing doesn't look that big. Could I have shrunk, or am I simply not as flexible as before? I'm a small woman and I remember having a little difficulty with my first boyfriend. Is this going to be like being 15 all over again—slowly stretching out the vagina until it's ready to fit something thicker than three fingers? I welcome your suggestions on how to play with my new toy.

There are several variables we must mention: What were the sizes of the penises you are remembering for comparison, how accurate is your memory, and whose three fingers is your standard for average width? (My gynecologist uses two rather slender ones as a guideline; maybe that's the difference between an optimist and a pessimist!) If none of your sex play over the past several years has included vaginal penetration of more than a finger or two, yes, it's probable that you've lost muscle tone and need to relearn how to accommodate more without discomfort. "Use it or lose it" doesn't mean forever, but it applies to toning muscles all over your body. Begin by using plenty of lubrication, on yourself and on the dildo, and try insertion when you are more highly aroused—perhaps just after you've climaxed by more familiar means. It won't take you long to accommodate your new toy, whatever its size.

My 25-year-old boyfriend of three years had his first homosexual experience at a very young age and has continued to have them as well as having relations with women. He has actually had many more male sexual partners than female. Since we've been together he's had about half-a-dozen brief gay encounters, using safe sex, he assures me. Besides this, he likes to dress like a girl sometimes and during sex pretend that we are lesbians. Usually he gets into cross-dressing when he is high, and when he is high is also the only time he will acknowledge his same-sex experiences. (When he's not high and I try to discuss this he gets angry, denies it all, and says he was just making up stories!) We have talked about getting married, but I have serious reservations. The transvestism doesn't bother me too much, although I'm curious as to what factors during the formative years would cause it. The real problem I have is dealing with the homosexual issue. It appears to me that he is dealing with a lot of guilt and repression because he seems to have two different personalities when it comes to his sexual orientation. I doubt that he'd agree to any kind of therapy, but even if I could persuade him to try it our funds are limited. Possibly you could suggest some books I could read to help me figure this out.

I agree with your take on the situation. Your man does sound troubled and I think your hesitations are well founded. Certainly you might make *mutual* exploration of some of these sexual issues a prerequisite to marriage by seeing a sex therapist together. That might feel a lot more supportive of your hopes for a jointly happy sex life than the inference that he needs to go get fixed before you'll marry him. As for books, you might start by browsing library copies of some good basics such as Kinsey's *Sexual Behavior In The Human Male*, or Shere Hite's more recent *Report On Male Sexuality*.

My girlfriend and I enjoy sex very much. To have an orgasm, however, she needs to have clitoral stimulation, and, well, blame it on bad engineering, that doesn't happen during intercourse. Someone suggested cock rings. The kind he recommended is made of

Ask Isadora

leather and loops smartly into a knot at the top—like the knuckle of a tightly-bent finger. This not only stimulates the clitoris during intercourse, but it also comes loose with a tug should things get too tight or uncomfortable. What do you think? Is the constriction of blood flow unhealthy? Are there other means of stimulating the clitoris during intercourse that you can recommend?

Anything that constricts blood flow too much or too long would be dangerous. (I would hope that the individual wearer would know what "too" was for him.) Since it would need to be quickly removable I would certainly avoid metal ones. I have never tried the leather ones you describe, but I have experienced leather rings with snaps—but no knots or knobbies—which I've seen worn by punk kids as wristlets. What you and I are discussing are French ticklers in the form of rings which go around the cock. For the sake of science my lover and I recently tried a rubber one. (Yes, yes, a dirty job, but...that's why being a sex educator is so much fun.) We bought it for less than $2 at an adult toy shop. It looked like a rubber soap saver with a hole in the middle and a protrusion at one end. With it slipped over the erect penis shaft like a "Do Not Disturb" sign over a door knob, it was possible to feel some added stimulation in certain intercourse positions, but not enough to provide anything really extraordinary for me. What it provided for him was a bruise over his pubic bone. Some folks swear by cock rings, however, and/or French ticklers, so if someone wants to write an Argument in Favor, I'm willing to consider it. Trying different intercourse positions and introducing your fingers, hers, or a vibrator will probably be more productive of orgasm during intercourse and have the added benefit of little if any discomfort for you.

Isadora Alman

I recently received a phone call on a weekend afternoon from a man saying he was doing a scientific research survey for "The Shere Hite Report." He sounded calm, legitimate and professional, so I answered the first series of questions regarding my sexual activities, fantasies and preferences. Gradually the questions became more personal, like asking me to touch various parts of my body as I described how it felt to be kissed there. When I expressed my discomfort, the researcher assured me he was a certified psychologist and that my responses would be confidential. The last question, he told me, was that I was to fantasize about my ideal partner, remove my clothes and masturbate to climax while he measured my breathing variations with some sort of instrument. Then I heard a click like a tape recorder. When I said "I can't do that!" he said "Okay" and hung up. Could this actually have been a legitimate survey method, or was this an obscene phone call as I now suspect? Since I gave out very personal information, I'm wondering if there is any place I can report this kind of call.

Can you believe that I got a call from the same creep? I said I would be happy to respond if he gave me his phone number so I might phone him back. When he of course refused, I let fly with some choice "judgments." Unfortunately, it is not a good idea to give out over the phone any information more personal than what radio station you're listening to. While there are many legitimate market researchers, there are just as many sickos and wrongos who can use such information in ways you would not approve. The phone company and the police will only concern themselves if you are subjected to repeated harassment. In your case, rest assured that most telephone thrill seekers like this one want only the instant high of an intimate conversation, often dialing at random until a cooperative woman answers.

chapter twelve
Resources and Research

Ask Isadora

As you know, the columns collected here were first published in *The San Francisco Bay Guardian*. When I wrote them I tried, wherever possible, to furnish local references and resources easily available to residents of the SF Bay Area. When putting together this collection, I wanted just the opposite—references and resources available nationwide, or a central contact for referrals to what is locally available elsewhere. When I had one, I rewrote my original answer. When I had no such handy answer, I simply omitted the question. What you have here then, are some resources you might avail yourself of wherever you are and *means* of finding out more about those which were mentioned in the columns on the previous pages.

This may be none of my business, but I'd like to know how you got interested in sex—professionally, I mean. I'm a psychology student and would like to know more about working in this field. Can you give me any leads?

There is no clear-cut certification for a "sex expert" like there is for a lawyer or journeyman steelworker. The term "sexologist" is still fairly new, and who qualifies as one is still open to interpretation and may vary from state to state. Several professional organizations such as The American Board of Sexology and The American Association of Sex Educators, Counselors and Therapists (AASECT), both based in Washington, D.C., do offer certifications. Other professional organizations for which there are membership qualifications are The Society For The Scientific Study of Sex (SSSS) based in Mt. Vernon, Iowa, and Sex Information and Education Council of the U.S. (SIECUS) in New York City. The members of their various local chapters are people-helpers of all kinds—medical personnel, counselors, teachers, or, in some cases, interested lay people (no pun intended). Few graduate schools offer advanced degrees in human sexuality. My own background is in psychology and communications. I became interested in sex, professionally, when I first took the San Francisco Sex Information Training for Volunteers. I still think it's one of the best programs I know of for those interested in communications, psychology, or sex. My experience on their volunteer phone line is the basis of an earlier book, *Aural Sex & Verbal Intercourse* (Down There Press).

Thank you for your open-minded treatment of the young man who found pleasure in wearing what our culture decrees are women's clothes. He is not alone! But most of us, especially of an older generation, must stay hidden. I hear that there are a few skirts for men being shown in high fashion New York boutiques. When do you think I will see a skirt on a male mannequin in Sears? A major torment in writing about this is being unable to give a return address for "off the air" communication. Like many hetero males of middle age who feel as I do, I would face social destruction if I revealed myself before the culture recognizes my activity as common. Is there an organization of like-minded hetero men and their women friends?

San Francisco's ETVC holds monthly social gatherings in a private meeting room and also conducts support and discussion groups for the female partners of participants. The group's purpose, says a spokesperson, is to demystify the activity and allow those interested or concerned to realize that people who enjoy cross dressing are just folks who, like cat fanciers or begonia cultivators, enjoy getting together to talk about

Ask Isadora

their common interests. If you write to the I.F.G.E. (International Foundation for Gender Education, P.O. Box 367, Wayland, MA 01778, they will let you know of a like-minded group near you.

I'm a single man of 22 without any sexual partner. Given the way things are today, it might be that way for a while. I'd like to know what sex toys are available for men and where to get them.

I spoke of several, like dildos, vibrators and shower nozzles in a recent *Bay Guardian* article on safe sex practices. There are a number of other enhancers as simple as creams and lotions for body stroking, or as complicated as a vacuum-like apparatus that sucks at the body part to which it is applied. It really depends on what you like or think might be fun to try. Consider browsing in an "adult" book store. There's at least one in every town, usually in its seamier section. Sexual pleasure items can be ordered from catalogs as well. Look for ads in sexually-oriented magazines like *Forum*. Two such catalogs are: Good Vibrations, 1210 Valencia St, San Francisco, CA 94110, and The Xandria Collection, P.O. Box 31039, San Francisco, CA 94131.

Are there any male sexual surrogates, and what do they do exactly?

There is an ancient one-liner that the definition of a mistress is somewhere between a mister and a mattress. A sexual surrogate is somewhere between a therapist and a lover in exactly the same sense. A good counselor or therapist will deal with such issues as shyness or sexual ignorance, verbally exploring with the client ways and means to overcome stumbling blocks to making an intimate connection. A good friend and lover will explore ways and means of making that happy intimate connection tailored expressly to the two of you. A good sexual surrogate, male or female, bridges the gap between verbal exploration of what pleasurable activities you might do with another human being and that time when you have a partner willing and able to do them with you. I call them "hands-on" therapists. IPSA Inc., The International Professional Surrogate Association (P.O. Box 74156, Los Angeles, CA 90004) might be able to connect you to a therapist in your area who refers to or works with surrogates.

A friend of mine was recently diagnosed with AIDS. Since he doesn't have any pressing medical needs at present, other friends and I are doing what we can to minister to his emotional needs by keeping him company as often as possible. Is there some sort of visiting volunteer corps like the home nursing services which exist for the physically ill that we might explore for those times when we're away this summer?

Cities and towns seem to do this on a local basis—sometimes through government funding, sometimes through religious institutions or hospitals, most often through grass roots support where there are politically active gay communities.

You have mentioned a drug used in cases of impotence, Papaverine. I would like to pass on to your readers some further information. My husband had become impotent as a consequence of diabetes which sometimes causes nerve damage resulting in an inability to achieve erection. Before we heard about the Pharmacologic Erection Program at University of California at Davis Medical Center, he was advised that the only solution for him was an implant operation which costs over

Ask Isadora

$5000 and is a fairly complicated medical procedure. The P.E.P. program is considered experimental. It cost only $700. There is a careful screening to determine that the impotence is a physical problem and that it can be helped with the drug, which is locally injected by the user. The P.E.P. program requires a commitment of regular visits, assessments, and follow-up over a six month period. Though it does not cure impotence, in most cases the use of this drug can restore normal sexual relations. The results for my husband have been very good.

Thank you for telling me about your good experience. Can we call this an "uplifting tale?" If Sacramento is not convenient to where you live, many local hospitals have similar potency clinics which offer alternatives to surgical implants. Call around, and be sure to speak to people who have gone through similar measures before making your decision.

I don't belong to a health club, so where else can I go to experience a real massage?

I'm going to assume that you're talking about a muscle-relaxing workout rather than a sexual experience when you say "real." Ads for masseurs and masseuses are ambiguous. Given current laws, they have to be. Look carefully at the wording in the phone book or newspapers. If pictures of some hunk or dolly are featured, if words like "erotic" or "sensual" are used, we can assume exactly that. (How "exactly" in some places, is up to negotiation.) If a particular style of massage is promoted, like shiatsu, or the ad says "non-sexual," it is likely that its intent is as described.

It seems that many women and men have had lovers try to convince them they should accept various forms of abusive treatment because "it's part of

S&M". Abuse is not a part of S&M. I belong to a group called The Society of Janus which advocates S&M as a valid sexual alternative as long as it is between adults, consensual, non-exploitive and safe. I have included one of the Society's cards and I would appreciate your giving them as a reference for anyone who wants to know more about S&M activities.

Done. A report in the Winter '87 edition of *The Journal of Sex Education & Therapy* states that "People who engage in S&M are usually motivated not by pain, but by dominance and submission. Most S&M'ers are aroused by the illusion of one person completely controlling—or being under the control of—another. Control, trust and fantasy are the central issues of S&M." The Society of Janus' card reads: "A non-profit organization which explores consensual Dominance/Submission, S&M, and Bondage and Discipline Relationships." For a potentially similar organization near you send a SASE to People Exchanging Power, P.O. Box 332, Edgewood, NM 87015.

Book Reviews and Gift Ideas

(Most toys, games and doodads mentioned here are available by mail from Good Vibrations Mail Order Catalog, 1210 Valencia Street, San Francisco, CA 94110, when not otherwise directed. Most books not obtainable through your neighborhood bookstore are also available from The Sexuality Library at the same address. Prices quoted, when they are, are approximate.)

Games Lovers Play: If it's a mild enough night to walk along the beach, or if you are fortunate enough to have access to a fireplace, judging from the romantic images of personal ad placers, probably little else is needed. If these are not

Ask Isadora

available, or more is required (beyond the basic requirement of a co-cuddler), here are some suggestions.

As a beginning to the evening's activities, or as a lead-in to a memorable end, borrow or buy *Enchanted Evening*. This is a board game for couples where players draw question cards eliciting—in the form of words or touches—revelations about sexual desires and daydreams. Unlike many other sex board games, this does not require expertise on the mating rituals of exotic fauna in order to win, nor impart culturally biased and often downright wrong "sex information." Sharing secrets under the guise of "following the rules of the game" is a painless path toward intimate connection ($20.)

A slightly more advanced game plan is offered in Kenneth Ray Stubb's and Louise-Andree Saulnier's book, *Romantic Interludes: A Sensuous Lovers' Guide*. This book provides instructions for sensual and sexual interactions, from ritual foot bathing to such erotic esoterica as "The Garden of Unearthly Delights," an activity which requires a selection of favorite foods.

For do-it-yourselfers, it takes no more than a pencil, paper, and a few minutes of private reverie to produce a list of questions and answers for you and your lover to exchange: "If I were your slave for one full hour, what would you have me do?" or "Pretend I am a prurient visitor from outer space and have never seen a human body. Take me on a verbal tour of yours, explaining in detail all its pleasurable aspects and functions."

Other materials for intimacy enhancement...or a plain old good time, are often readily available. An exchange of massages can be a simple, and simply delightful affair, without the necessity of a special table or odoriferous oils. A painter's drop cloth of treated paper or plastic is available for no more than fifty cents through building supply stores. Kitchen-variety corn starch provides a silky sensual texture to clean, dry skin, and is much easier to vacuum out of your bed or carpet. If you prefer a slicker texture, compressed coconut oil (available in health food stores) is inexpensive, edible, and melts very obligingly under the heat of eager hands. If the massage recipient (and taking turns is quite in order) is blindfolded to better allow for tactile experiences, you won't believe the wondrous sensations which can be produced by trailing a silk tie or scarf, a fur ear muff, a feather duster, a paint brush, or gently-held bath scrubber slowly along the length of a body.

* * *

• Any intimate conversation, whether verbal or non, is likely to be enhanced by musical accompaniments of your favorite record or tape. (A favorite of mine is a collection of underground blues numbers from the '20s and '30s called *Copulatin' Rhythm*, produced by Jass Records, Box 689, Greenport, N.Y. 11944.)

> Penises are cute but they're not logical
> Don't let them make decisions for you
> I think penises are wonderful
> I like to play with them
> Masturbation is loads of fun
> And so is loving other men
> Watch them grow before your eyes
> Lie back and watch them shrink
> They can do a lot of things
> But don't use them to think!
> Don't use your penis for a brain

Ask Isadora

> Hard as it may be, you really must refrain
> Cause it's meant to bring you pleasure
> But it's bound to bring you pain
> If you try to use your penis for a brain.

The lyrics excerpted above are by Ron Romanovsky (published by Bodacious Music, ©1986, Fresh Fruit Records, 2269 Market Street #301, San Francisco, CA 94114). If you are not familiar with the work of Romanovsky and his partner Paul Phillips, you're missing a treat. Some of their other poetic and musical gems are entitled "Wimp" ("I hate to bother you, but would you mind if I sang this song. I'm sorry, you probably aren't interested...") and "What Kind Of Self-Respecting Faggot Am I?"—a lament from a man who neither reads *GQ* nor owns any records by Barbra, Bette or Judy.

• Every year or so, *Condom Sense* has occasional updates of its bright, witty and informative newspaper on that very subject—condoms, how to choose them, how to use them, and other pertinent commentary ($2 to P.O. Box 30564, Oakland, CA 95604).

• An old favorite book of mine is Dorothy Tennov's *Love & Limerence: The Experience of Being In Love* (Scarborough Book edition, Stein & Day Publishers, 1981, $7.95, softcover). This book will appeal to people-helping professionals as well as lay persons, lovers, would-be-lovers, and never-have-been-in-lovers who want to understand what all the fuss is about. Psychologist Albert Ellis' cover quote reads: "An unusually profound and yet down-to-earth and useful discussion of the state of being 'madly' in love. Fascinating reading!" A few books in each generation define and direct the development of a new branch of science. This book does just that for psychology and sexology.

Isadora Alman

- *Erotic Communication,* by Natalie and Ralph Bacon (Shakti Press, P.O. Box 2249, Berkely, CA 94702, 1985, $9.95, softcover), is about Ralph, a 74-year-old widower with erection problems who through a personal ad meets Natalie, a 59-year-old non-orgasmic former lesbian. They fall in love, get married, have lots and lots of sex and presumably live happily ever after.

I find this book valuable on many levels. While tell-all autobiographies of the rich and famous gush tales of who does what sexually with whom, seldom do we ever get to know what goes on in the bedrooms of people who might be very like ourselves. Also, this book does much to dispel myths—myths of too old, too ill, too set in my ways, too late, too anything for good sex.

- Joani Blank, sex educator and proprietor of Good Vibrations in San Francisco, is also the author of three delightfully different stocking stuffers: *The Playbook For Women About Sex* ($4.00), *The Playbook For Men About Sex* ($4.00), and *The Playbook For Kids About Sex* ($4.75), available from Down There Press, P.O. Box 2086, Burlingame, CA 94010. Include $1.00 for shipping and handling.

These play—as opposed to *work*—books are cleverly drawn and hand-lettered exercises in looking at personal attitudes and myths about sex. Gently, and with humor, the reader is encouraged to check multiple choice boxes, complete sentences, draw pictures, compose ads and write stories on such topics as—how I feel about my body, exactly what is sexually arousing to me, how I feel about women and about men and communicating with myself and others. All of these three books are non-fattening, non-threatening, inexpensive, educational and fun. They can be enjoyed in private or enjoyably shared.

Ask Isadora

Now could you say the same thing about whatever this year's equivalent is of the hula hoop?

• *How They Do It,* by Robert A. Wallace, (Wm. Morrow & Co., 1980, $4.95, paperback), is a book I often read from on my radio program. The author, a zoologist with extensive background in the social systems of animals, is not only knowledgeable, but an extremely entertaining writer as well. Witness his account of a porcupine in rut displaying his erection: "As if this behavior weren't crass enough, when he gets within six or seven feet of [the female], he begins to drench her with short spurts of urine (a good trick in itself, since not many mammals can urinate with an erection, and six feet is not bad in any case). This unchivalrous soaking can be a bit much for her and she may amble away, perhaps to think through the entire matter one more time."

This is a marvelous book for young science students or their prurient parents. It not only covers thoroughly and delightfully the birds and the bees, but everything else from bacteria to bats.

• *Ultimate Pleasure: The Secrets of Easily Orgasmic Women,* by Marc and Judith Meshorer (St. Martin's Press, 1986, $14.50, softcover). My father used to say that complements are like perfume—you can't pass one along without having some of the lovely essence stay with you. Giving this book to an important woman in your life will definitely reap benefits for the giver. This is not a how-to book exactly, more like an unsung "I did it my way." Several sexually responsive women tell their stories, how they think and feel and what they do. The backgrounds and perspectives of the women interviewed vary enormously. If there is one theme common to most, it's one readers of "Ask Isadora" will be familiar with—know yourself and communicate that knowledge. This is an important book for women, and the people who relate sexually to them.

• Some columns back we discussed how to educate oneself or a partner in the joyous art of oral sex. I have received resource recommendations from several readers. One is *The Ultimate Kiss*, by Jacqueline and Steven Franklin (L.A.: Media Publications). Another is a Warner paperback, *The Intimate Kiss*, by G. Legman (Is that a misplaced namefreak, or what?). And still another: *The Joys of Oral Love* (B.J. Hurwood, Ed., Carlyle Communications, 1975). A final recommendation is a hilarious book I would give a substantial body part to have written myself, Cynthia Heimel's *Sex Tips For Girls* (Simon & Schuster, 205 pps, $7.95). One of many suggested inducements to use on a reluctant muff diver: "Next time you're walking down the street and spot a veritable Adonis, point to him and say, "Isn't Marcello over there amazing? You'd never guess that he's actually sixty-seven years old, would you? The doctors were baffled, but then they found out that there is a certain youth-prolonging enzyme secreted by the vagina which, mysteriously enough, can be absorbed only by pressing the tongue directly on the clitoris. And the more you move the tongue in light, flicking motions, the more of this enzyme is absorbed into the bloodstream. Marcello's been lapping up this enzyme for years."

• As a gift for an intimate, or he or she you would like to have as such, may I suggest Safe Sex Gift Arrangements available from Exodus Trust, 1523 Franklin St., San Francisco, CA 94109.

Ask Isadora

Collections of condoms, lubricants, lotions and hard-to-find latex novelties like gloves and rubber dams are prettily arranged in willow baskets and heart-shaped boxes priced from $4 to $30. You could, of course, assemble something like this on your own, but why buck the shopping throngs? Use the time you save to bake some cookies to accompany your basket of goodies.

• Now would be a good time to (re)discover the wonderful wisdom of Virginia Satir. Particularly for parents, but for anyone who ever had them, *Peoplemaking*, originally published in 1972 and updated in newer editions, is a good place to start. See your neighborhood library or bookseller.

• Aptly-named Down There Press, those wonderful folks who brought you (ahem) such gems as *Aural Sex & Verbal Intercourse* by yours truly, has published *Herotica*, a collection of women's erotic writings. There is something for everyone here.

• Beg borrow or steal a copy of *The Two-Step: The Dance Toward Intimacy*, written by Eileen McCann and illustrated by Douglas Shannon (Grove Press, 1985, $9.95, paperback). This book of cartoons says much more about how it is between men and women (and any other combination, actually) than many a mighty tome I've waded through. Two other books just out on your favorite subject and mine which are worth reading are *Intimate Matters: A History of Sexuality In America*, by John D'Emilio and Estelle Freedman (Harper & Row, $24.95, hardcover), and *Erotic By Nature* (Red Alder Books, Box 2992, Santa Cruz, CA 95060, $35 plus postage), which is a collection of fine-quality erotic photographs, writing and drawings by and for women and men.

Isadora Alman

Reported tidbits from various professional sexologist conventions:

• There are three major aspects of any disability that may affect sexual functioning—medical (injury, malformations, consequences of surgery, effects of medications), functional (pain, fatigue, paralysis), and psychosocial (incorrect beliefs, anxiety, depression). Many of the sexual problems confronted by disabled individuals and their partners are related less to the physical impairment itself than to the feelings and often erroneous beliefs about it "Looking like this, who could want me now?" "I would love to hold him/her, but I'm afraid it would hurt."). Some ways out of these binds: Focus on potentials rather than what is impaired. Adjust medication dosage and timing to provide maximum control of symptoms when sexual activity is desired. Learn more. Become educated to allow for more realistic expectations. Talk about specific fears and possible solutions with health care givers, others with the same condition, family, friends and lovers. Redefine sex as more than genital intercourse—an excellent idea for us all. (From a presentation by Julie Botvin Madorsky, M.D., Pomona, CA, recently honored as National Physician of the Year.)

• Pleasure does more for you than create smile crinkles around your eyes. It also releases endorphins which, among other good things, enhances the immune system. Sex being one of life's greatest pleasures when it works right, here are some ways to keep the activity levels up in long term relationships: Don't attempt intercourse before passion rises (through talk, fondling, mutual disclosing, sharing a sense of the illicit). Dress for sex in whatever little embellishments turn your partner on (costumes, lingerie). Develop and enhance all of the senses (paying attention to a particular contour of the lover's body; getting into what has been a turnoff, like caressing a scar or bouncing on excess body weight; smell and sniff and use scents; play music; make sounds; feed each other; play-act). Recapture a feeling of high arousal: re-enact your first time, dress in prom clothes, have sex outdoors. Remember, there is a thin line between embarrassment and excitement. (From a presentation by Stella Resnick, Ph.D.)

• Rape conjures up horrifying images of a stranger leaping from behind bushes to grab a perfectly sober unsuspecting woman whose dress and demeanor are in no way provocative, and through violence and threats of violence forces her into sexual acts. But if, for instance, the rapist and his victim dated, or if she was flirting with him in a bar beforehand, or in fact she went home with him but decided after some fondling and fumbling that she didn't want to have intercourse and he begged or bullied her into it—in other words, the further any specific incident deviates from the picture as originally painted, the less likely either of the people involved, much less a jury, is likely to perceive what happened as rape, *although it was*. By law, rapes are divided into two categories—aggravated rape is a situation in which someone is threatened, force or violence is used, the victim is attacked by more than one rapist and/or another crime is committed at the same time. Simple rape involves no force or violence, simply a sexual act to which consent was not freely or legally able to be given. Therefore, a woman who is shamed and taunted into giving in with "Whatsamatta, you frigid or something?", or a *man* who gives sex

Isadora Alman

because his boss implies that a promotion might go with it, has been raped. So has the wife who is "doing her duty" or the "willing" young woman of 17 here in California. It is not uncommon, then, for someone to be unsure whether she/he has been raped, or for a person to refuse to see he has committed one. Some men have been known to phone the woman they have left sobbing on the floor and ask for another date! Lest you think the topic irrelevant to your life, earlier this month the United Press International wire carried a story on a survey of 1,700 junior high school students in which half the boys and 41% of the girls said a man has the right to force a woman to kiss him if he has spent 'a lot of money' on her (which these 12-year-olds defined as $10 to $15). (From presentations by Bernard Apfelbaum, Ph.D of Berkeley's Sex Therapy Group, and Andrea Parrot, Ph.D. from Cornell University.)

• Two key factors in the cause of what used to be called premature ejaculation (but may less judgmentally be termed "eager" or "early"—ejaculating before one wants to) are a combination of high arousal state and performance anxiety. There is no quick fix to this condition, but there are methods of gradually building control by focusing on the pleasure and comfort of sex rather than a specific goal. Communication skills are vital since the man must be able to ask for his partner's cooperation in what is, after all, affecting both people. While improvement is common, a caution here is that a natural sprinter is unlikely to turn into a marathon runner no matter how much training he does. In one timed study men identified as early ejaculators came two-and-a-half to three minutes earlier, even during unhurried solitary masturbation, than men

Ask Isadora

who did not report having a problem. The partners of early ejaculators are urged to not fix blame, be warm and affectionate, but not to say intercourse doesn't matter when it does. Learn to avoid fights caused by sexual tension and to enjoy other forms of sexual expression and affection. And, partners, less you feel unloved and unlovable, remember, "You didn't cause the problem and you can't fix it." (From separate presentations by Drs. Barry W. McCarthy, Donald S. Strassberg and Nicholas S. Aradi.)

• In a study of couples married happily for more than 25 years, their sleep patterns and other biological rhythms were remarkably similar. Cause or effect, who knows?

• Each of us is exposed to approximately 400 ads a day—TV, radio, magazines, newspapers, billboards—on the topics of love and sex. Two-thirds of the songs in the Top 40 at any given time echo those themes. One billion dollars is spent every hour in the United States on cosmetics. Do you suppose there is a correlation?

• A questionnaire given to 200 middle class married Floridians turned up the following fact: the more these couples had sex, the more exciting they found it. (It occurs to me that the reverse is far more likely to be true.) One of the key ingredients in making it more exciting for women was "sexy clothes," and for men, X-rated films. Both partners found changing the customary times, places and positions of marital sex also spiced things up.

• When physical testing devices are used, (many) women turn out to be equally aroused as (most) men by viewing sexually explicit material, but often they do not know that this is so. They either block out their body's signals of excitation or have never learned to recognize them.

• In the almost inevitable power struggle

Isadora Alman

which occurs within every couple, she or he with the least power often shows the least desire for sex. (Remember the typical marriage image of the '50s? Harriet Housewife always has a headache.) In dependency struggles (who needs whom more) the stronger partner usually demonstrates less interest in sexual activity.

- In letting the audience of sex educators know what we were up against, Faye Wattleton, President of Planned Parenthood Federation of America, told us of some of the teaching methods of the "Just Say No" Chastity Brigade. You know, those folks who are sure that keeping your legs crossed will cure all the ills of the world. When beset by temptations of the flesh, concupiscent teenagers are urged to "pet your dog instead of your date" and "pretend you're on a date with Jesus." (Actually, I find this an incredibly hot fantasy, but then, if I weren't perverse, would I be in this business?)

- According to research by Richard Grant, M.D. for 52 couples seeking sex counseling, issues of sexual dysfunction were interrelated with relationship issues. (I find that almost invariably true in my own counseling practice.) If both partners report sexual problems, he says, they are more likely to stay in therapy than when the identified problem is the male's alone. (I, for one, fail to see how a sexual problem within a couple can belong only to one person.)

- Jack Morin, using questionnaires about individuals' most exciting experiences and fantasies, postulates four psychological "cornerstones" as the basis for eroticism: 1.) violation of prohibition (given our society's sanction for little beyond heterosexual married missionary procreative intercourse, that one's a cinch), 2.) longing (you know, the lure of the unattainable and

"Always leave 'em wanting more," 3.) the quest for power ("Honey, I love to make you moan and groan"), and 4.) ambivalence about intimacy (remember how ol' Erica Jong spoke to the secret places in all of us when she first wrote of the zipless fuck?)

• Stella Resnick, who promulgates "sex without sex" (I prefer the term "outercourse"), defined intimacy as congruence between what's going on inside and what is allowed to show outside. While acknowledging that much of the open discussions on topics once not even spoken about in whispers is embarrassing for many people, she suggests relabeling those feelings of embarrassment. Think of those flaming cheeks and pounding heart as manifestations of arousal, which they are, and enjoy. Use the laughter of tension to lighten up. Embarrassment can be sexually stimulating. She quoted a profound piece of wisdom by that old philosopher George Burns: "The secret of happiness is being happy."

• Dr. Joe Wells, in a delightful study of sexual terminology, found that while heterosexual men and women and lesbians "make love," gay men prefer to fuck. When using specifically erotic terms as a turn-on, heterosexual men and women speak different language, the women preferring euphemisms or clinical terms such as "fondle" or "penis," while straight men prefer slang such as "jack-off" or "dick." Since they don't like the same terms, it's no wonder that heterosexuals use them less with their lovers than do lesbians and gay men. By the way, while some may talk of "genitals" and others of "cocks and cunts", gay men do not report having any erotic term for female genitals. Pity!

• Preliminary studies by Dr. David Quadragno seem to give some support to the belief that young men more often seek sexual intercourse for physical reasons and young women for emotional ones. However, at or about midlife, the trend seems to reverse itself. All the more reason, say I, for we who are mellowed and matured, to match up with the young'ns.

- Research by Brian Gladue (wherein he paid college students to look at erotic photographs: "A dirty job...") seems to support a long-held belief of mine that while some people get aroused by perceived danger, for many women feeling "safe"—however they define that to themselves—is a prerequisite for feeling sexual.

- HIV status, + or -, is showing up more and more as a pertinent fact in gay men's personal ads.

- Private studies indicate major differences between condom brands as to strength, stretchability and effectiveness of protection. Until those studies are published and names are named, change brands if you're having trouble and use water-based lubricants with Nonoxynol-9 (*not* baby oil, *not* hand cream). Mineral oil destroys latex within 60 seconds of contact! And while 75% of men ejaculate within two minutes of initiating sex (not intercourse; this statistic includes "foreplay"), that still leaves you about a minute with that condom in jeopardy.

- Author Carol Cassell acknowledges the ambivalence of the modern woman who hums "I Am Woman, Hear Me Roar" in the morning and "Someone To Watch Over Me" at night. She says what women want is "a Three-S Man"—sensitive to her needs, supportive of her work, and successful in his work. When questioned by an audience member about a fourth, sexy, Dr. Cassell said that if a man meets the requirements of the first three he will automatically be considered as the fourth.

Ask Isadora

(I discussed her proposition on my radio show that evening and got agreement from several callers that such criteria are non-gender-specific nor necessarily sexual. Who wouldn't want as a friend someone who met that description?)

• Dr. Herbert Otto emphasized how little our culture knows about such an important topic as the orgasm. (Every supermarket magazine is ballyhooing the clitoris as if it were a new washday miracle, yet some women climax from back rubs and neck kisses. While Masters and Johnson insist that all orgasms are alike, More University is teaching classes on how to have one that's more than an hour long. Dr. Dean Edell says female ejaculation is a myth and Dr. Beverly Whipple shows movies of several women spurting like Old Faithful. Let's get together on this, folks, and recognize the enormous spectrum of possibilities.) He says that differing orgasm kinds and strengths and lengths and causes are culturally programmed, limited only by our beliefs about what we are capable of. More research is needed. Okay, reader, pick your favorite topic and do some research.

Ask Isadora

About the Author:

Since February, 1985 *The San Francisco Bay Guardian*, an alternative paper with the largest circulation of any newsweekly in Northern California, has been running Isadora Alman's extremely popular column on relationships. On the right-hand side of the continent, the *New York Press* has carried her column since 1989. Readers' queries have run the gamut, from the standard "Where can I meet (...solvent men/willing women/swinging groups)?" to such esoterica as an effective way to suck toes. Isadora's answers are to the point and often funny, pertinent not only to the San Francisco Bay area or greater New York City, but to anyone hip-deep in the delights and dilemmas of creating intimate connections in this perplexing world.

Addressing the question of whether sex could be construed as aerobic exercise, she responded: "Most health and fitness purists would probably say not...but since it requires no designer costumery, little in the way of equipment expenses, and usually a minimum of travel to arrive at the site of the sporting event, I say 'Go for the burn!'"

To the man who wanted to know what to do about his sensitive nipples: "Say to whomever might find this of interest, 'My nipples are extremely sensitive, so please do (or do not, according to your preference) touch (stroke, fondle, nibble, pinch) them.' Or, place (or remove) hands and mouths which wander near, again according to your preference. If your partners are anywhere as sensitive as your nipples, they will soon get the picture."

Isadora Alman has been called a hip Dr.

Isadora Alman

Ruth, a sexy Dear Abby, and a bawdy Miss Manners. She is the author of a book, *Aural Sex & Verbal Intercourse*, published in two languages; has for many years had her own weekly call-in radio show; and has lectured widely on communication skills and sexuality. Her counseling practice is in San Francisco. It just might be time for men and women outside a few metropolitan areas to become familiar with the broad range and universal applicability of her wit and wisdom.